FOOD
COMBINING
FOR HEALTH

D0111691

FOOD COMBINING FOR HEALTH

Doris Grant & Jean Joice
Foreward by Sir John Mills C.B.E.

Illustrated by Rita Greer

THORSONS PUBLISHERS, INC.
ROCHESTER, VERMONT
WELLINGBOROUGH, NORTHAMPTONSHIRE

Thorsons Publishers, Inc.
One Park Street
Rochester, Vermont 05767

First published 1984

© DORIS GRANT AND JEAN JOICE 1984
© JOHN MILLS 1984

© DORIS GRANT AND JEAN JOICE 1987
© JOHN MILLS 1987

sle

Library of Congress Cataloging in Publication Data

Grant Doris.
  Food combining for health.

  Bibliography: P.
  Includes Index.
  1. Health 2. Nutrition. 3. Cookery (natural foods)
4. Proteins – metabolism. 5. Carbohydrates – metabolism.
6. Hay, William Howard, 1866–1940.
I. Joice, Jean. II. Title.
RA784.G72 1985   613.2   84-26822
ISBN 0-7225-0882-4

Printed and bound in the United States

10 9 8 7 6 5 4 3 2 1

Distributed to the book trade in the United States by Harper and Row

Distributed to the book trade in Canada by Book Center, Inc., Montreal, Quebec

Distributed to the health food trade in Canada by Alive Books, Toronto and Vancouver

Cover design by Ann Aspell

CONTENTS

PART THREE: RECIPES FOR PROTEIN MEALS

PART FOUR: RECIPES FOR STARCH MEALS

ACKNOWLEDGMENTS

We would like to thank Dr. Jeannie Stirrat for so tirelessly extracting for us, during the past seven years, many pertinent and helpful items from her medical journals and papers.

We would also like to thank Mrs. Gordon Clemetson, Dr. John Breakwell, and Dr. Hugh Cox for taking the time to read this book in manuscript and for their continuing interest and encouragement.

Our gratitude is owed to the editors of the *Hay System News* of the 1930's for much valuable material, and to the editors of *Healthy Living* and *Here's Health* for publishing Doris Grant's articles on the Hay System; it was the enormous interest these created that prompted the writing of this book.

Finally, we would like to thank Pamela Kelly for her immense patience in typing and retyping the many amendments to the recipes, and Anthea Gordon for producing an impeccably consistent manuscript from two very different styles.

FOREWORD

by Sir John Mills

I am delighted to know that the Hay Diet is being resuscitated after all these years. I have a copy of the original book, which my sister, Annette, gave me over forty years ago, and on the flyleaf is written "John Mills' Bible. Please do not remove."

In 1942 I was invalided out of the Army with a man-sized duodenal ulcer. In hospital I was fed on the usual ulcer-sufferer's diet of rice puddings, mashed potatoes, and so on, and after three months, there was no improvement. In fact, I became a walking zombie.

My sister, Annette, suggested to my wife, Mary, that she should put me immediately onto the Hay Diet, and my first meal, which I remember with gratitude, was a thin minute steak, a large mixed salad, and a small glass of dry red wine. From that moment I have never looked back. After six weeks, I was able to start work on a film.

Most diets, I find, are crashing bores, especially to hostesses, but if one follows the Hay Diet, it is possible to go to any dinner, public or private, and offend no one. All one has to remember is the principle of not mixing starch with protein. So one can wade one's way happily through any festive occasion until it comes to the dessert. I find the best way of coping with this is to leave the dessert untouched, and the waiter will finally remove it, and nobody will have noticed.

I am sure that I could not, at my advanced age, cope with the work I have on hand at the moment if I were not a "believer." I am playing eight shows a week in *Little Lies* at Wyndham's Theatre, and the last Act is a marathon. It is essential that I am really fit, and for this I rely practically entirely on the Hay Diet. I am, incidentally, today wearing the jacket that I had made for me in 1938. It has not been let out, and I can still button it without any problem.

I wish the book every success, and I guarantee that anyone who follows the advice in it will derive the greatest of benefits from it.

INTRODUCTION

A Personal Experience

As we eat even so are we; our health is made or marred with our feet under the dinner table.

This fundamental truth was forcibly brought home to me in my late twenties, when a severely painful attack of rheumatoid trouble in my joints suddenly took all the pleasure out of my life. When the usual medical therapies had been applied, with no effect whatsoever, a doctor-cousin came to the rescue with an unorthodox medical prescription. It consisted of three columns of foods—proteins, starches, and acid fruits—accompanied with the instruction: "Don't mix foods that fight!"

By the end of just one week, this unusual prescription, conscientiously carried out, produced a totally unexpected bonus: the complete termination of nagging indigestion pains of fifteen years' duration.

By the end of just two weeks, there were more unexpected results: an ability to think more clearly than before and a great general feeling of well-being, which inspired me to carry on.

By the end of four weeks, all the rheumatoid pains had gone and have never returned.

By the end of a year, I felt like a new woman. I was tireless and filled with a new energy never before experienced. The more difficult the task the more I welcomed it as a challenge to my newly found health and abilities. Yet apart from not eating meat or acid fruits (apples, oranges, pears, grapefruit, and so on) with bread and sugary foods at the same meal, there had been no other change in my diet. And this still included white bread and refined sugar, to whose potential dangers for health I had not then been alerted. This fact is of the highest significance; it provided unique evidence that "not mixing foods that fight" really works.

Toward the end of the first year of compatible eating, I discovered and studied Dr. William Howard Hay's inspiring book *A New Health Era*, and found that there was much more to compatible eating than "not mixing foods that fight."

As a result of reading this book, my diet and health improved still further; I felt that I had set out on a marvelous adventure. I must admit, however, that departing from my usual eating habits was not at first a rose-strewn path. Relatives and friends, especially medical friends, pooh-poohed the idea of any connection between food and health, and thought that I had taken leave of my senses, whereas, in fact, I was just beginning to come to them. Friends argued that I was going to miss out on all the joys of eating: "What, no sugar? No crackers and cheese? No apple pie?—you *poor* thing!"

I found, however, that food is much more enjoyable when it is the right kind—fresh, whole, unprocessed, and properly combined. Moreover, by cutting down sugar and eventually cutting it out entirely, my taste buds became much keener and I began to enjoy delicious, new gastronomic experiences. In no sense was this a "diet" to follow for a short time, or a temporary cure for a specific condition. Rather it was a philosophy of living, involving a return to properly constituted foods and common sense principles, which ensure health and fitness, and minimize the necessity for medical treatment.

The fitter I became the more convinced I was that *we hold our health in our own hands, to a very large extent.*

By the end of four years of compatible eating, I produced a much longed-for second child *nine years after my first-born,* despite warnings from my doctor and a gynecologist after the first birth that *I could never have any more children;* there had been serious complications after an emergency Caesarian operation. But they had not reckoned with the healing powers of compatible eating! Moreover, the second birth according to the gynecologist, was a "textbook demonstration of a beautifully normal birth"!

By the end of another three years, I had collected abundant proof of these healing powers while writing long weekly articles on the Hay System for a well-known national Sunday newspaper—the now defunct *Sunday Graphic*—in 1936 and 1937. These articles continued for nine months and generated enormous interest, bringing into the *Graphic* office hundreds of letters every week.

The letters were an education, and most revealing; their almost monotonous single message was the complete failure of medical treatment as far as the degenerative diseases were concerned; the "wonder drugs" never effected the hoped-for cure. Often there were recitals of complete disaster in treatment, and of the "cure" being far worse than the disease, frequently proving fatal.

As the weeks and months passed, however, there were many accounts, from followers of the articles, of greatly improved health, benefits often being felt even within the first week. There were also reports of increased zest for living; depression replaced by optimism; digestion pains eliminated; freedom from colds; arthritic pains lessened and freer movement; and constipation a thing of the past. Many readers reported great relief from tiredness and chronic sleeplessness. One unforgettable letter was from a woman of seventy who wrote: "I feel well for the first time in my life!"

These letters provided convincing proof of Dr. Hay's contention: that the primary cause of disease is not the outside germ, which always gets the blame, but the inside state of the body, created mainly by wrong living habits and wrong eating habits.

The *Graphic* articles soon brought Dr. Hay to London. His objective was to ask me to write a book of menus and recipes for the Hay System, adapted to the needs of the British housewife. This I did. Before returning to the US after a successful lecture tour in England, he reviewed the book and gave it his blessing. Unfortunately, it is now out of print – hence the present book. We hope that this new look at the Hay System will stimulate fresh interest in a way of eating that has such tremendous potential for health and healing.

DORIS GRANT

PART ONE

THE THEORY AND THE PROOF

by

Doris Grant

1.

A GREAT PIONEER

William Howard Hay was born in Hartstown, Pennsylvania, in 1866. Prophet, philosopher, hard pan Presbyterian of Scottish stock, he grew up from early boyhood with the sole thought of medicine as his calling.

He was fortunate that both his parents were of exceptional character; his father, according to Dr. Hay, "was possessed of an unusually fine mind, was a great reader of good literature and developed into one of the solid men of his community." His mother "combined with a very excellent education the Scottish characteristics of thrift and industry, with also one of the most even dispositions imaginable, an ability to see through a great many things that looked difficult to others, and a sense of right and wrong that knew absolutely no compromise." Dr. Hay was richly endowed with his parents' fine characteristics, and these undoubtedly provided him with the courage and strength of character to overcome the heartbreaking difficulties that beset him when his unorthodox treatment of disease evoked the enmity of his colleagues.

He graduated from the University of New York on March 26, 1891. For the next sixteen years, he practiced medicine "according to the best light of his time." At the end of this period, his health began to deteriorate, proving, as he admitted, "that he knew as little as the rest of the predisposing causes of disease." He became very ill, developed

Bright's disease, high blood pressure, and finally a dilated heart. For this latter condition, medical relief was only temporary. He thought his career was over, and his doctors warned him to put his affairs in order.

Inspiration
In *A New Health Era*, Dr. Hay related how this warning inspired him to treat his own symptoms. He did so by "eating fundamentally," as he called it, eating "only such things as he believed were intended by nature as food for man, taking them in natural form, and in quantities no greater than seemed necessary for his present need." (It is interesting to note that sixty years later, T.L. Cleave was to put forward similar concepts in his book *The Saccharine Disease*.) To the great astonishment of Dr. Hay's doctors, his symptoms gradually disappeared, and at the end of three months, he felt fitter and stronger than he had for many years. He reduced his weight from 225 lbs to 175 lbs and soon was able to run long distances without distress.

This experience, he wrote, deepened his conviction, which had been growing over the past sixteen years, *that medicine was on the wrong track*; it was merely fussing with the end results of a condition instead of attempting to remove the cause, "for here was his own case recovering from a condition that the best authorities said was incurable." A major health disaster and a hopeless outlook for the future opened his eyes to the possibility of treating disease through diet, unorthodox as this at first seemed.

It was not, however, till the middle of 1908 that he had recovered to his own satisfaction. By 1911 Dr. Hay was virtually certain that he had discovered a "sure-fire treatment" for diabetes. He little realized then that this same treatment would prove equally efficacious in the treatment of all diseases.

For the next four years, he devoted all his time to treating his patients through diet in order to prove or disprove his contention that we are exactly what we eat and "that the body is merely a composite of what goes into it daily in the form of food and drink." Those four years provided proof in plenty that his contention was right and that anyone can be as well as desired if given the right food in the right way (provided, of course, there has been no serious, irreversible organic change). Thus he developed over the years the system of eating for which he became famous. He always claimed, however, that *he had not discovered anything new*, but had merely used the knowledge already made public by others and consolidated it, adding his own deep convictions with a dash of common sense. Moreover, he made no claims that he "cured" any disease, and emphasized that this system merely removed the obstacles in the way of nature's own marvelous healing powers.

The message in *A New Health Era* was simple: that no matter how diverse our diseases, they have one underlying cause—wrong chemical conditions in the body. These conditions are created through the manufacture and accumulation of the acid end-products of digestion and metabolism in amounts greater than the body can eliminate. A condition then develops "that is variously called autointoxication, acid-autotoxicosis, toxemia, self-poisoning, or whatever you like to call it." This results in a lowering of the body's vital alkaline reserve, leading in turn to departure from health. "The science of medicine takes no cognizance of this accumulation," wrote Dr. Hay, "till disease—that is, definite pathology—has developed."

He taught his patients that there were four main causes of the accumulation of the acid end-products of digestion: eating too much meat; overconsumption of refined carbohydrates—white flour products, refined sugar, and refined carbohydrates of any kind; disregard for the laws of chemistry as these apply to the digestion of foods; and constipation.

Dr. Hay also taught his patients that although many people, especially young people, build up a tolerance to incompatible mixtures, just as people build up a tolerance for increasing doses of irritant poisons, they do so at considerable and continuing cost in vitality. This tolerance, he

warned, is unnatural. But if compatible eating is followed
long enough, it can be removed. Then, claimed Dr. Hay,
"you cannot go back to the practice of mixing starches and
proteins without immediate notice from your stomach that
you have made a mistake—one that you are not likely to
repeat." He promised that two weeks would be sufficient
to convince anyone of this, and that the reward for the effort would be greatly improved vitality and health.

Dr. Hay never forgot to teach the importance of other aids
to health—fresh air, exercise, daily baths, sunshine, and rest.
Nor did he forget to teach the importance of health to the
spiritual man: "When the body and mind are in harmony,
only then will there be an opportunity for proper spiritual
development; for do not forget that the spiritual man is the
first man, the mental man the second, and the physical the
third man; and only when these second and third are in
harmony, can there be a proper spiritual state."

Disbelief
In spite of the ease and speed with which people could
prove for themselves the truth of the starch-protein concept, the Hay System received a barrage of criticism.

The bitterest attacks came from Dr. Hay's fellow physicians. Teaching the means of preventing disease had not,
in Dr. Hay's time, caught on with the medical profession,
simply because their entire teaching had been (and still is)
directed towards the *treatment* of disease, not its *prevention*.
Dr. Hay's teaching was therefore stark heresy and was naturally condemned as such.

As he became more and more convinced of the truth of
his findings, so his colleagues became more and more skep-
tical. Ironically, while realizing success in his treatment of
disease beyond his wildest hopes, restoring to normal health
countless cases termed hopeless by the highest of medical
authorities, he found himself written off as a quack. His frus-
tration must have been immense when, armed not only with
an inspired idea but also with proof of its truth, he was met
with a wall of disbelief and incomprehension.

The medical profession was most certainly not ready for Dr. Hay's concepts. At that time, doctors were fervent apostles of "the germ theory of disease." They were also enthusiastic about the new wonder-drug era, which promised "a pill for every ill"; so they believed that there was no need whatsoever for nutritional therapy. His concepts were rejected with scorn, and he was constantly subjected to the vehement opposition of entrenched orthodoxy, and even to slander, libel, and the most vicious of rumors. But he was a courageous man who never faltered in defending his beliefs and in countering all opposition with lucid and reasoned arguments, never losing his temper or his strong sense of humor. The latter attribute, and his great personal charm, endeared him to his patients and to all who had the good fortune to hear him lecture.

It is significant that many physicians attended his lectures in both England and Scotland, and many of these spoke to Dr. Hay afterwards and said they were in full accord with everything he taught. Some admitted that they were students of the Hay System and were using it in their work with their patients. Many, moreover, told of results that could not have been achieved in any other way, except by applying the system with real understanding.

Dr. Hay died in 1940, at the age of seventy-four, a year after a serious accident. Sadly, he died just as medical thinking was beginning to appreciate the important relationship of nutrition to health.

Vindication
That Dr. Hay was "a prophet way ahead of his time" has now been fully confirmed by the vast change in attitudes toward nutrition by many of the foremost medical authorities in both the US and Great Britain. Despite all the marvels of modern medicine, despite the wonder drugs and the astronomical cost of our health services, the health of both nations is deteriorating and disease is attacking at an increasingly early age. Medical authorities are now frankly admitting that medicine is on the wrong track and they are

urging a switch of emphasis from curative medicine to preventive medicine—to dealing with the *causes* of disease instead of merely treating *the symptoms*. As a result, nutrition is now being promoted as the first priority in preventive medicine. In fact, attention is now being focused as never before on the close relationship between nutrition and health, *and on just such concepts as were held sixty years ago by Dr. William Howard Hay, gifted surgeon and general practitioner of note.* Witness the following signs and portents:

- Since the 1950s, the research and writings on human ecology by a number of medical scientists have produced evidence of the close connection between refined carbohydrates and chemically adulterated foods and such diverse symptoms as allergies, depression, migraine, fatigue, skin diseases, schizophrenia, and uncontrolled aggressive behavior in children. The research, in particular, of Dr. Théron Randolph and Dr. Ben Feingold in the US, and of Dr. Richard Mackarness in Great Britain, has been outstanding. They are nevertheless fighting the same bitter battle for recognition by orthodox medicine as did Dr. Hay fifty years ago.

- A society formed in Great Britain in 1967, The McCarrison Society, whose members consist of doctors, surgeons, dentists, veterinary surgeons, and community health workers, is pledged "to advance education in, and initiate, carry out, and sponsor, research into the relationship between nutrition and health. . . ." The society was named after the internationally acclaimed British nutrition pioneer, the late Sir Robert McCarrison, whose book *Nutrition and Health* should be mandatory reading for all health-conscious people. Dr. Hay claimed that he owed much to McCarrison's teachings.

- In 1968, the validity of the germ theory of disease was seriously questioned for the first time in a leading British medical journal. In *The Lancet* of May 18, Professor G.T. Stewart revealed its weaknesses in a revolutionary paper "Dogma Disputed, Limitations of the Germ Theory." Stewart's message was, in effect, that acceptance of the germ theory as the main cause of infectious disease has been responsible for orthodox medicine overlooking other more important, or equally important, causes such as genetic and metabolic effects, behavior (smoking and so on), and *certain nutritional deficiencies.*

- In the 1970s, Cleave's epoch-making book, *The Saccharine Disease,* started the present revolutionary medical preoccupation with bran and "fiber," nutrition, and preventive medicine. It postulated one common cause of many of the present-day degenerative diseases—the consumption of *refined carbohydrates.* Moreover, it has become the major reference work for the growing number of medical specialists throughout the world who believe—as Dr. Hay did—that our twentieth-century diet is responsible for today's vast number of diseases.

- Also in the 1970s, another important book, *The Role of Medicine: Dream, Mirage or Nemesis* by Professor Thomas McKeown, contained the blunt message that more attention should be paid to nutrition, and that the modifications of the conditions which lead to disease will achieve more than any medical intervention after the illness has begun. That, too, was Dr. Hay's message.

- In 1972 the Editor of the *British Medical Journal* exhorted: "We now have to learn the more subtle relationships that exist between nutrition and medicine, and how change in food habits and change in methods of food preparation may affect health. *Medical education must keep pace with the rapid advance in this subject."*

- In 1977, this same Editor wrote: "Enthusiasm for fiber is sweeping the world. The journals are full of it, the popular press revels in it, and doctors take time off from prescribing it only to attend international conferences on it . . . in 'discovering' fiber, modern man is waking up to the fact that his food is systematically deprived of fiber on its journey from field to grocery shop."

- Also in 1977, the Editor of *The Lancet* stated: "About five years ago, dietary fiber burst into the consciousness of the medical world, having smouldered at the back of some minds for decades."

- In 1981, the magazine *Which?* (the British equivalent of *Consumer Reports*) discovered in its researches that more people than ever are clamoring for drugless treatment. (This, however, is not sufficient — people must also be willing to *assume responsibility for keeping themselves fit*.)

- In 1982, on December 14, at the British Medical Association's 150th Annual Dinner, Prince Charles affirmed, in his presidential speech, with reference to drugs: "Wonderful as many of them are, it should be more widely stressed by doctors that the health of human beings is so often determined by their behavior, their food, and the nature of their environment."

- In January 1983, in *Homeopathy Today*, a doctor wrote that he advised his patients "not to eat high proteins with high carbohydrate foods," and stressed the importance to health of recognizing the trinity of mind, body, and spirit.

- Also in 1983, remarkably, the potential for health of "fringe medicine," now elevated to the status of "alternative medicine," was being considered by a new research committee. *Hospital Doctor* of April 14 reported that "alternative medicine" was to be "put under the scientific spotlight" by the Research Council for Complementary Medicine, which would consist of both conventional and alternative specialists. This Council had been formed "because of growing public interest in acupuncture, homeopathy, and herbalism." The committee believed that it could "help to stop the erosion of public confidence in orthodox medicine."

- Finally, in June 1983, in his speech on stepping down as president of the British Medical Association (BMA), Prince

Charles urged: "Don't overestimate the sophisticated approach to medicine. It seems that account has to be taken of those sometimes long-neglected complementary methods of medicine."

It appears that his message had the desired effect. On August 17, 1983, the British press announced that in a revolutionary move, the BMA was launching an inquiry into all forms of alternative medicine and that some may soon become available from the British National Health Service. In the *Daily Mail* John Illman wrote: "The move marks a remarkable about-face for the BMA, which for years has resisted what has been regarded as "quack medicine" . . . the background to the BMA move is the growing interest in Britain in health matters and preventive measures against illness."

In this same article, Illman quoted Dr. Malcolm Carruthers, author of *The Western Way of Death*: "There is a crisis of confidence in drugs. No medical system can afford not to take account of the public's desire to play a larger part in determining their own medical treatment."

Illman also quoted Dr. Anthony Fry, consultant physician in psychological medicine at Guy's Hospital: "As a profession we have spent too much time giving Valium instead of teaching patients how to relax. *We spend too much time treating symptoms and not causes.*" So affirmed Dr. Hay, sixty years ahead of his time, throughout all his writings.

What better vindication could this prophet have than the decision of the BMA to launch an inquiry into alternative medicine?

A New Health Era
It appears from these "signs and portents" that the "new health era" so dear to Dr. Hay's heart has indeed begun. If this book contributes to this era, even in a small way, by helping its readers to achieve greater health and happiness, its authors will perhaps have repaid a small part of the great debt they both owe Dr. Hay for countless benefits received

from his teachings. How better to end this chapter than in his own words:

> To really live is to be in exuberant health continually, and when in that condition nothing palls on one, nothing is devoid of interest, and life is the swellest job in the world. When in splendid health, every breath we draw is filled with inspiration, everything we do is full of interest; there are so many things to do, so much to accomplish, so many delectable prospects in life that even if we are poor and unknown, we still may fully enjoy life, for life is a splendid thing if we are really alive.

2.

THE HAY SYSTEM EXPLAINED

There is nothing so powerful as an idea whose time has come

The Hay System consists of five important rules:

1. Starches and sugars should not be eaten with proteins and acid fruits at the same meal.
2. Vegetables, salads, and fruits should form the major part of the diet.
3. Proteins, starches, and fats should be eaten in small quantities.
4. Only whole grain and unprocessed starches should be used, and all refined processed foods should be taboo—in particular, white flour and sugar and all foods made with them, and highly processed fats such as margarine.
5. An interval of at least four to four-and-a-half hours should elapse between meals of different character.

The cardinal rule of the Hay System—not mixing carbohydrates (i.e., starches and sugars) with proteins and acid fruits—is generally misunderstood, although based on sound physiological principles, long existing and long forgotten. In order to understand this rule, it is necessary to understand the classification of carbohydrates and proteins in the context of compatible food combinations:

1. *The proteins* are concentrated (20 percent or more) animal proteins such as meat, fish, cheese, and poultry.

2. *The carbohydrates* are concentrated (20 percent or more) starches, such as grains, bread and cereals, potatoes, and sugars.

A misunderstanding regarding this classification has been the main reason why many investigators have dismissed the starch-protein concept as being without foundation. The main argument put forward to refute this concept is that nature herself combines proteins and starches in most foods; that if it is wrong to combine these dissimilar elements at the same meal, then nature herself is in error.

On first glance, this argument seems unanswerable; it is widely acknowledged that nature does not make mistakes.

On second glance, this argument reveals shallow thinking; nature does not combine in one food *a high concentration* of protein (as in meat) with *a high concentration* of starch (as in grains). Although meats do contain a carbohydrate, it is in the form of glycogen, which requires little, if any, digestion, and its presence therefore does not interfere with the conditions necessary for protein digestion. Similarly, although grains contain about 10 percent protein, this is an incomplete protein, and is not in a concentrated form (as in meat); its presence therefore does not interfere with the conditions necessary for starch digestion.

Apart from the single exception of mature, or dried, legumes—peas, beans, lentils, and peanuts—nature combines starches and proteins in the same food in a form and in proportions that digest together perfectly, and in such a way, also, that the food is either predominantly starch or predominantly protein. The dried legumes are "the exception which proves the rule"; they contain too high a percentage of both protein and starch to be compatible in themselves (but become compatible and highly beneficial when sprouted—see Part Two, "The Hay System in Practice"). People who are accustomed to the habitual consumption of legumes over a long period can build up a tolerance to them. But people who are not accustomed to them usually experience discomfort—and audible protests from their digestive organs!

The Why and How of Starch and Protein Digestion
Proteins require an acid medium for digestion. When animal proteins enter the stomach, this stimulates the production of hydrochloric acid, which activates the enzyme pepsin, whose function is the splitting and digesting of the proteins. This action in the stomach can only take place in a wholly acid medium; the presence of any high starch or sugar, with its accompanying alkalies, interferes with, or neutralizes, this acid medium, and the proteins are then incompletely digested. The implications of this incomplete protein digestion are more serious than has hitherto been suspected. This is discussed in Chapter 3, in relation to allergy.

Carbohydrates (starches and sugars) require an alkaline medium for digestion. This is initiated in the mouth by the action of ptyalin, an enzyme that splits the starches into lower forms before they enter the small intestine, where their further reduction *and main digestion* take place. As the whole process of starch digestion depends on its proper initiation in the mouth, all starchy foods must be thoroughly chewed; otherwise the small intestine, though alkaline in all its secretions, cannot complete what the ptyalin started higher up in the tract.

The stomach acts as a mixing chamber in which the saliva, with its active ptyalin, is thoroughly incorporated into the starches. During this early sojourn in the stomach, lasting about thirty to forty-five minutes, the normal acidity of the stomach is insufficient to cancel out, or interfere with, the alkaline medium necessary for preparing the starches for their intestinal digestion. The presence of meat, however, or other acid-inducing foods, or acid fruits, arrests this preparation, and fermentation follows; the splitting process of starches can only occur in a positive alkalinity.

When asked what was the scientific basis for the theory that starches and sugars should not be eaten with proteins and acid fruits at the same meal, Dr. Hay replied:

> If starches are taken combined with acid fruits, and if the stomach contents are withdrawn at intervals during digestion, it will be observed that the action of ptyalin has ceased and that the starches are not being split but will give the intense blue reaction of iodide of starch when iodine is applied to the chyme removed from the stomach. The same test may be performed with a combination of starches and proteins – the extraction of parts of chyme at intervals, as they happen during our digestion, will always show this arrest of ptyalin digestion, meaning that the starches then unsplit will never be properly split.

For many years, the teaching has been that the highest levels of acidity are in the resting stomach. This belief has been responsible for the advice given year after year, and still given to ulcer sufferers, "to avoid letting the stomach get empty." But a number of authorities disagree with this belief (now in disrepute in certain medical quarters), including the physiologist A.H. James. In *Physiology of Gastric Digestion*, he states: "The highest acidities of all are reached *during the digestion of food, not when the stomach is empty.*"

This fact supports Dr. Hay's contention that if no protein accompanies a starch food entering a resting stomach, the amount of hydrochloric acid is insufficient *at first* to fully neutralize or overcome the alkalinity of the saliva present.

In 1936, the work of three Philadelphia investigators provided interesting laboratory confirmation of the starch-protein concept. In *Man Alive, You're Half Dead!*, Dr. Daniel Munro gave an account of a study of five subjects by the investigators, showing the degree of acidity in the stomach after protein meals, after starch meals, and after combined protein and starch meals. This study revealed that one and a quarter hours after these meals were eaten the stomach contents were most acid after the high protein meal, least acid after the high starch meal, and half way between both states after the mixed meal. Moreover, when the mixed meal was eaten, it was clear that the proteins were being digested with difficulty. The acidity present was far lower than that required by the all-protein meal and had actually been cut by one-third by the presence of the starches and their accompanying alkalis.

This investigation clearly showed that when high starches and high proteins are mixed at one meal, there is too much acid to permit the continued alkaline reduction of the starch part, and not enough acid to start the digestion of the protein part.

The usual teaching, however, is that when we eat food *of any kind* (such as proteins and starches) we produce gastric juice, which contains hydrochloric acid. The answer, here, is that hydrochloric acid is stimulated in exact ratio to the amount of protein presented to the digestive task. This was shown by Ivan Pavlov's classic observations on dogs in *The Work of the Digestive Glands*.

As already pointed out, the protein in starches such as grains is both very small (about 10 percent) and incomplete, and therefore does not stimulate sufficient hydrochloric acid to interfere, *for the first thirty to forty-five minutes,* with the alkaline medium necessary for the digestion of starches. During this time, the saliva—which has a pH value of 6.6, as compared with the pH 0.9 of pure gastric juice—acts as a natural buffer to the gastric acid.

Some physiologists and physicians disagree with Dr. Hay's explanation of the starch-protein theory and claim that the gastric acid is *necessary* for the splitting of the starches; the starch is often contained in protein "envelopes" that require the acid for digestion so that the starch can be released. This claim is undoubtedly correct but it does not alter the fact that starches have a preliminary digestion in an *alkaline* medium, which buffers the gastric acid for the first thirty to forty minutes in the stomach. There is, therefore, still plenty of time for the gastric acid to work on the starches during the remaining three or more hours that they are in the stomach before entering the small intestine. There, of course, the pancreatic juice completes the digestion of carbohydrates (starch, dextrin, and the like), and also of protein, in a mainly alkaline medium.

Whether Dr. Hay's theory is right or wrong, however, does not really matter; the indisputable fact remains that his theory most certainly works. As he pointed out, any doctor who claims that it does not has never given it a fair trial; otherwise he could not with honesty make such a claim.

The Importance of the Chemical Balance

For optimum health and heightened resistance to disease, the diet should, ideally, consist of alkaline-forming foods and acid-forming foods in the ratio, approximately, of four to one, which, when metabolized, will produce a corresponding ratio in the body.

When Dr. Hay was asked what was the scientific basis for this ratio, he replied:

> We have no way of arriving at the relative proportion of alkaline and acid elements needed by the body except through an analysis of its excretions. When we take into account all of the excretions through the four avenues of elimination, we find that the loss in alkali is four times as great as that in acid. This means that if we would replace our losses fully we need four times as much of the alkaline intake as of the acid intake. This is a fact well known to physiologists and can be verified in almost any work on physiology.

With regard to the chemical balance of the human blood, Dr. Hay wrote:

> It may seem strange that the slight difference between a pH 7.1 and 7.6 spells the wide difference between an acidosis and an alkalosis, yet this is true; and even this slight variation makes all the difference between function of the most chaotic variety and that of high efficiency.

Judging by the average of those of his patients who had conserved their alkaline reserve for several years through observing the proper ratio of alkaline-forming foods to acid-forming ones, the "normal" alkalinity—as distinct from the "average" one—should not be much below pH 7.5. From the standpoint of *averages*, this is considered an alkalosis, yet when the alkalinity of the blood is sufficiently high to show pH 7.5, "there is extremely high functional activity, with comparable feeling of good health, mental activity and physical efficiency."

Another interesting and important light is thrown on this question of alkalinity by Dr. Dudley d'Auvergne Wright in *Foods for Health and Healing*. He points out that "the normal alkalinity of the body fluids is the most favorable one for the action of vitamins."

It is not difficult to distinguish between alkali-forming and acid-forming foods:

1. *Alkali-forming foods* comprise all vegetables (including potatoes, if cooked in their skins and the skins are eaten); all salads; all fresh fruits (except plums and cranberries); almonds; and milk.

2. *Acid-forming foods* comprise all animal proteins such as meat, fish, shellfish, eggs, cheese, and poultry; nuts (except almonds); all the starch foods such as grains, bread, flour, and other foods made from cereal starches; and sugars.

Complete lists of both types of foods are given in the Appendix.

It should be emphasized at this point that there is sometimes confusion for some people regarding the classification of "acid" fruits (grapefruit, oranges, lemons, berries, and so on) as "alkaline-forming." This classification does *not* relate to the "acid" taste of the fruit but to its *end-product* in the body. The acid fruits, moreover, are the foods that deposit the highest alkaline ash of all foods. It is an interesting fact that the acids of these fruits leave the body within an hour or so of being eaten. They do so via the lungs (mainly), and the skin, urinary tract, and bowel. The alkalis,

when released from their combination with the acids, provide a highly valuable contribution to the body's alkaline
reserve. The only way in which acid fruits can be said to
be "acid-forming" is when they are wrongly combined with
starches at the same meal, when they can cause an uncom-
fortably full feeling, or even pain. Sufferers then conclude
that acid fruits don't suit them!

In order to approximate the ideal four-to-one alkali-acid
ratio, the day's meals should include one protein meal only,
one starch meal only, and one wholly alkaline meal, with
occasionally two, or even three wholly alkaline-forming
meals. An occasional "health day" on nothing but frequent
meals of one kind of fruit – a *gesundheitstag* as it is called in
Germany – is highly beneficial. Young children and people
who do a lot of manual work can, however, require extra
starch meals. How to plan these meals is described in Part
Two, "The Hay System in Practice."

A word of warning is necessary here. To opt out of the eating habits of the herd does require, at first, a certain amount
of self-discipline. For this reason, compatible eating is not
recommended for people who are content with their state
of health, or who can eat incompatible mixtures without discomfort or apparent harm. Dr. Hay warned that some
people do not have the essential "burning desire" to improve their health, or the will-power to see the thing
through. He therefore advised that any change in the diet
should be made slowly, by degrees. It is quite sufficient,
to begin with, he said, just to observe the starch-protein
rule. When this change is well established, the natural whole
foods – especially those in uncooked, salad form – should
be gradually increased, and any refined carbohydrates, and
other processed foods, should be proportionately decreased.

The number of alkaline-forming meals should then be increased. Especially recommended, when starting the diet,
are vegetable or salad meals containing delicious potato
dishes; they are not only less expensive but also more satisfying, in a cold climate than meals of only vegetables, salads,
or fruit.

Compatible eating, it should be pointed out, can be as cheap—or as expensive—as the budget allows. And it is definitely more economical, as small correctly combined meals are better digested and thus more satisfying than large incompatible combinations; it is not *the amount* of food that counts, but *the amount that is properly digested, absorbed, and metabolized by the body.* Proof of this fact for followers of the Hay System is the fading desire for between meal snacks. In these days of soaring food prices, *more nourishment for less food deserves serious consideration.*

It is important to note that observing the rules for compatible eating considerably reduces the amount of fats in the diet, especially those fats arbitrarily occurring in so many processed, supermarket foods today—and this reduction takes place despite the culinary use of cream, which raises compatible eating to delicious heights of enjoyment. Cream, in moderation, is almost a necessity for this way of eating. *Healthwise*, there is no cause for concern as explained in Chapter 4 "Animal Fats—Fact and Fiction." *Costwise*, the extra expense of cream is balanced by the savings that compatible eating makes possible on other foods such as expensive, ready-made, "instant" foods and meat.

It is even more important to note that observing the rules for compatible eating *automatically reduces* the acid-forming foods in the diet and *automatically increases* the alkaline-forming foods that are rich in accessory food factors, thereby contributing to the alkaline reserve and a well-balanced body chemistry. In this correct chemical balance lies the secret of health and resistance to disease.

An interesting analogy, here, is provided by the fact that the correct alkali-acid balance is also of importance in the soil. In the *Soil Association Journal* of December 1973, Michael Blake draws attention to this fact and stresses that the effect of an imbalance is not restricted to the soil, but is of "universal importance to all living organisms."

Finally, it cannot be repeated too often that the Hay System is not a joyless, wearisome "diet" but a "philosophy of living." A new convert, Joan Hodgson, enthusiastically agrees. In *A White Eagle Lodge Book of Health and Healing*, she writes:

> Harmonious food combining is a way of life. Once the rules have become familiar, imaginative cooks can have fun thinking up the most delicious meals. This is not a régime of constant self-denial, but of rethinking the meals so that each one is based on family favorites, with food combined in such a way that more nourishment can be extracted with less tax on the digestion, and consequently more energy for enjoying life.

Fifty years of "enjoying life" on the Hay System, and the experience gained in helping countless people to regain health by its means, have convinced me that health is our normal state, that we were designed, created, and born to be healthy. This experience has also provided abundant proof that correct eating can not only greatly improve the quality of life but can also prevent many of the degenerative diseases.

3.
THE HAY SYSTEM AND THE DEGENERATIVE DISEASES

The hope of humanity lies in the prevention of degenerative and mental diseases, not in the care of their symptoms.

Dr. Alexis Carrel

There is a generally held belief today that people are living longer than before. Although more children survive to reach adult life, middle-aged people have scarcely improved on the life expectancy of their great-grandparents. The unpleasant truth is that, instead of living longer to a healthy and enjoyable old age, we are merely taking longer to die.

Moreover, with each generation, there is an increase in the ordinary diseases of degeneration, and these are appearing at ever earlier ages. All the "tremendous new discoveries" in the drug field have been unable to stop this increase. Belief in the curative power of drugs has contributed to this increase by diverting attention from the positive promotion of health.

As a result, the disillusioned medicine prescribers and medicine takers are now showing a healthy interest in the doctrine of "holism" — treating whole people rather than just their disease symptoms. This is completely in line with Dr. Hay's common-sense principles, which more than ever before are shown to be valid. He advocated the treatment of patients themselves — not their symptoms — and argued that it was childish in the extreme to suppose that we can restore people to full health without first rooting out the cause of their diseases; to do otherwise was just as stupid as bailing out a leaky boat without first finding and stopping the leak.

Dr. Hay also argued that the cause, in every case, is the same thing—*food* (overconsumption of refined carbohydrates, and incompatible combinations). The degenerative diseases are just different manifestations of this one cause. The cure, he pointed out, "therefore lies in food always and only."

This *unitary concept of disease* bears a close resemblance to that advocated by Cleave in *The Saccharine Disease* (except regarding incompatible combinations, with which Cleave was not in accord). He, too, indicts *food* (overconsumption of refined carbohydrate) as the cause of disease and he, too, points out that the degenerative diseases are just different manifestations of this one cause. This concept, known as "the saccharine disease" (i.e., relating to sugar), is now grudgingly conceded by the medical establishment, and enthusiastically accepted by a growing number of doctors internationally.

Among these manifestations, Cleave listed *constipation*, with its complications of varicose veins and hemorrhoids; *obesity; diabetes; skin diseases; dental decay* and *periodontal disease; urinary tract infections* (such as cystitis, from which so many women suffer today); and *coronary disease*. Dr. Hay dealt with most of these manifestations and others as well, but nowhere in his many writings have I found any reference whatsoever to coronary heart disease (CHD).

This fact is highly significant; it confirms Cleave's contention that it "takes *time* for the consumption of refined carbohydrates to produce the various manifestations of the saccharine disease," and that these manifestations have "incubating periods" that differ in each case. In the case of diabetes, for instance, the incubation period may be twenty years, but in the case of CHD, thirty years. As CHD was a rare disease from 1900 to 1930 when Dr. Hay was practicing medicine, it is not surprising that he never had to deal with it. It was still a rare disease in the 1920s and it was not until thirty years afterward, in the 1950s, that CHD started to become an epidemic, *concurrent with the massively increasing consumption of refined sugar.*

CHD incidence in the West is now among the highest in the world. In 1983, 38 percent of all deaths in the US were attributable to heart disease, and in 1985, 43 million Americans had one or more forms of heart or blood vessel disease.

Doctors admit that the causes of CHD are not known with any certainty, and that they are still ignorant of its dietary requirements. But on BBC-TV in June 1983, in a series of programs called "A Plague of Hearts," a new approach to preventing it was advocated by a leading epidemiologist, Professor Geoffrey Rose—the creation of *"a more healthy lifestyle for the whole population."*

Dr. Hay also advocated this approach—not for CHD, which was virtually nonexistent in his lifetime, but for treating and preventing *all* degenerative diseases. There are a number of very good nutritional "cures" now being promoted, but it can be stated categorically that the Hay System comes nearer to a full understanding of the causes, treatment, and prevention of disease than any other doctrine, as the following discussions of some of these degenerative diseases will confirm.

Constipation (simple)

Fifty years ago Dr. Hay listed constipation as one of the main sources of acid formation in the system and warned that, if long continued, it could be the cause of many of the degenerative diseases. Present-day medical findings have confirmed this warning and have also revealed that constipation is almost certainly a contributing factor to the high rate of bowel cancer in advanced nations.

Dr. Hay also listed incompatible food combinations and fiber-deficient refined carbohydrates as sources of acid formation. Both these sources directly contribute to constipation. Striking proof that they do so was provided in a paper entitled "Amylaceous Dyspepsia" (starch-caused indigestion), published in *The Liverpool Medico-Chirurgical Journal* in 1931. Its author was Dr. Lionel J. Picton, author-in-chief of the famous *Cheshire Medical Testament*, published in 1938, in which thirty-one family doctors declared that *the prevention of sickness depends on correct feeding.*

In this paper, Dr. Picton drew attention to a well-known laboratory experiment on dogs by the famous Russian scientist, Ivan Pavlov. From this experiment, according to Picton, Pavlov deduced the following data: minced beef fed to a dog is digested in about four hours; starch by itself passed through a dog's stomach in a much shorter time — in one-and-a-half hours or less — white bread passing more slowly than brown. *But when meat was mixed with the starch, there was invariably a delay — a protracted delay.* Instead of the four hours for meat alone, this mixture took eight or more hours to leave the stomach.

Picton argued that this delay in one section of the digestive line indicated delay all along the line. As he pointed out, "The somewhat startling conclusion flows from this, that meals of mixed character such as meat and bread favor constipation, whereas meat and salad at one meal and starchy food such as bread and butter at a separate meal have no such effect."

Picton's paper provided outstanding confirmation of the truth of the starch-protein concept, and of the close relationship of incompatible food mixtures to constipation. And his case histories of patients provided proof.

The first step in the treatment of constipation is therefore none other than that recommended by Dr. Hay for all diseases, *the removal of the cause* — far too much acid-forming meat and carbohydrates (especially refined carbohydrates), far too little alkaline-forming vegetables, salads, and fruits, *and incompatible food mixtures.* Instructions for "the removal of the cause" are given in Part Two, "The Hay System in Practice"; they are not difficult to follow and will in fact *simplify* meal-planning, and lessen the time spent cooking and the costs of cooking.

No matter how correctly meals are combined, the fiber in the diet should always be increased by taking unprocessed wheat bran daily. It should be taken at first in teaspoon doses, in water, before meals, increasing gradually to suit individual needs. Dr. Neil S. Painter, a well-known London surgeon, advises: "You are eating enough bran only when you can pass soft stools without straining. Once you have found this amount, take it for life." Recent research has shown that in western countries, the daily stool is hard and viscous compared to that of rural Africans and Asians living on unrefined foods, and that the intestinal transit time may be as long as *five* days instead of twenty-four hours. Thus, many people who think that they are not constipated may be very constipated indeed, *despite having a daily bowel movement.* For this reason, and in order to speed recovery from *any* disease, Dr. Hay suggested taking a daily two-quart, cool, plain water enema, but not without professional instruction.

Indigestion (standard type—upper abdominal pain, heartburn, sometimes accompanied by acid regurgitation) This is a condition that for many people has become an accepted evil and part of their lives. It is most frequently caused by treacherous food mixtures and it responds with astonishing rapidity to compatibly combined ones. I have rescued many people from the afternoon indigestion pains that can result from lunchtime sandwiches of bread and cheese, or bread and meat. They all marveled at the ensuing peace and tranquillity in their interiors!

In *Peptic Ulcer,* Cleave argues that the main cause of indigestion is eating refined carbohydrates which are stripped of protein, resulting in an outpouring of gastric secretion where there is not enough protein to neutralize it. This argument, however, is somewhat difficult to reconcile with the fact that, in spite of eating refined carbohydrates (white bread and sugar) during my entire first year of compatible eating, I nevertheless lost indigestion of fifteen years' duration during the very first week.

Dr. Hay, too, was convinced that in many, perhaps most, cases of indigestion, refined carbohydrates were the cause, but for a different reason. Picton was likewise convinced. In the aforementioned paper, he stated that his evidence for this conviction was "mainly clinical," having found that reduction of refined starchy food intake relieved his patients' symptoms. For "the incipient dyspeptic," Picton recommended "a diet in which more greens and grilled meat should replace some of the bad foods of modern times, and moreover a diet in which starchy foods should be separated as far as possible from meat, and taken at separate meals"—a diet totally in accord with Dr. Hay's precepts.

Naturopath Harry Benjamin also believes that combinations of starch and protein foods can cause digestive trouble. In *Your Diet in Health and Disease,* he recommends cutting out bread and potatoes with meat.

Dr. Hay warned that taking antacids, the patent "cure" for indigestion is not the answer; they can compound the trouble, leading to more serious conditions. There have been medical warnings today that antacids can use up certain vitamins in the body which are vitally necessary for its proper functioning. Moreover, experiments at Cornell University, revealed that administering carbonate of soda and milk caused a form of kidney stones in laboratory animals. Antacids are merely a crutch that deals with *the symptom instead of the cause.* The best treatment for indigestion is compatible eating.

Arthritis

The cause and cure of arthritis, whether rheumatoid or osteoarthritis, has baffled the medical profession. Doctors frankly admit as much; they prescribe anti-inflammatory drugs and painkillers, and tell their patients they must learn to live with their disease. The side effects of the painkillers, however, can be serious, even lethal, as the effects of one "wonder drug" for arthritis, Opren—now withdrawn— proved all too tragically. "No drug to date has cured, or ever will cure, a true case of arthritis," wrote Dr. Hay.

There are many contributing causes of arthritis, such as injuries, abuse of the body, allergic reactions, infections, stress-exhausted adrenal glands, vitamin D deficiency, and so on. But the end result of most of the underlying causes produces one common denominator—deranged body chemistry. A main cause is therefore an accumulation of acid end products of digestion, resulting in a lowered reserve of the alkaline buffer salts. Dr. Hay stressed that "the function of every organ and tissue depends on the height, breadth, and depth of the alkaline reserve; and the lower this is the lower the function. . . ."

The logical approach to treatment is therefore a nutritional one, aimed at the deranged body chemistry and *not at the joints* as in the conventional drug and surgical treatments presently in vogue. These are merely palliatives that, once again, deal with the symptoms instead of grappling with the causes.

In a personal communication, Dr. James Lambert Mount, author of *Food and Health of Western Man* and one of the founders of the McCarrison Society, described how he had successfully applied a nutritional approach when treating a hundred volunteer patients, suffering from arthritis, who took part in an experiment in New Zealand. They were put on *a diet aimed at changing the body from an acid to an alkaline state,* by giving up red meat, flour, and sugar, and concentrating on salads, fruits, and organ meats. There was an average 80 percent success rate, varying from considerable improvement in the arthritic condition to a complete cure.

Arthritis is considered the least amenable to treatment of all the chronic diseases. But Dr. Hay maintained that arthritis responds to nutritional treatment as surely as do other degenerative diseases. Twenty-eight years of experience enabled him to write very positively—and comfortingly—about the ultimate cure of arthritis:

> Most cases of arthritis are curable, and permanently so, if the disease has not progressed to such a degree that it has permanently destroyed the function of the affected joint as occurs in ankylosis. As long as there is motion left in any joint, the case is by no means hopeless. Do not be discouraged if the pain seems to inhibit motion completely, if at the same time the joint can be moved passively to any degree.

He warned, however, that deposits outside the circulation, such as those in the tissues about the joints, may require years to be completely absorbed or may never be fully absorbed, even though the joints may become usable and pliable, without pain. But he promised that even cases of severe arthritis, where every joint in the body is painful and immobile, will recover uniformly when the body is relieved of its excessive debris and feeding is corrected.

He said that no specific diet is necessary, or even advisable, for arthritis, but it is essential that the food intake be largely of the alkaline or base-forming variety—vegetables, salads, fruits—and be kept so throughout life; that the colon should be brought up to date (i.e., the bowels emptied) and kept so. It is essential that the diet should contain fresh, properly constituted foods, whole foods, and *as much as possible of these in raw form*. It is interesting that, in 1936, at the Royal Free Hospital in London, an experiment on arthritic patients with a raw diet was successfully carried out by Dr. Dorothy C. Hare. In the report of this experiment in the *Proceedings of the Royal Society of Medicine* (Vol. 30, 1936), Hare stressed the fact that the raw state of the food seemed to be the one outstanding factor that brought about results.

Dr. Hay warned that starches and sugar—carbohydrates of concentrated character—are the chief dietary causes of arthritis, not so much because they are so intrinsically causative, as because they are usually eaten in combination with incompatible foods and their proper digestion is prevented, with resulting fermentation.

The elimination of starches and sugar in the diet is therefore of paramount importance. In the opinion of some authorities at the present time, most arthritic patients experience difficulty in assimilating carbohydrates, with ensuing indigestion. (Once again, starch is the villain, and even a valuable whole grain one can be so if not correctly combined with other foods). From my own experience and that of correspondents and friends, indigestion frequently precedes and accompanies arthritis. This indicates that both conditions are due to the same cause—incompatible food mixtures and a lowered alkaline reserve. This underlines the great value of compatible eating; it automatically reduces the amount of starch eaten and ensures its compatible combination with other foods.

Many of Dr. Hay's patients recovered fully by making no other dietary change apart from the strict separation of incompatible foods (as in my own case). But to make this strict separation and, at the same time, make the diet 80 percent alkaline-forming, is more effective, more speedy, and more helpful in correcting the chemical balance. Arthritis, asserted Dr.Hay, is a purely nutritional state, the result of an imbalance in the body's chemistry; he found this evident from the observation of many cases. He also found it evident that "exposure to weather, or occupational pursuits, have nothing to do with the creation of the condition, except in a secondary way."

To help correct the chemical balance and increase the delicate alkaline reserve in the blood-stream, Dr. Hay particularly recommended acid fruits such as oranges, grapefruit, and lemons (the juice of a lemon in a glass of water on waking is very beneficial); these acid fruits are especially high in alkaline salts—lemons most of all. Unfortunately, many arthritic sufferers make the mistake of avoiding all "acid fruits" thinking thereby to help their condition, whereas they are merely worsening an already deficient intake of vitamins. As there seems to be much confusion regarding the term "acid fruits", the reader is urged to reread its classification in Chapter Two, "The Hay System Explained."

Dr. Hay also recommended:

• Celery juice. This has proved invaluable in dissolving and removing years of accumulated acid deposits in the cartilage of arthritic joints. In *The Home Herbal*, Barbara Griggs recommended celery seeds for arthritis and rheumatism because their "high alkaline value helps to counteract acid formation in the blood and clear it out of the system." Arthritis sufferers will find her other recommendations very helpful.

- Wheat germ, bran, kelp (seaweed, obtainable in tablet form at health food stores), and *cod liver oil*. Dr. Hay claimed that these supplements are also very beneficial for *all* departures from health.

- *Gentle exercise, rest,* and *natural sunlight.* Research by Dr. John Ott, famous pioneer of time-lapse photography, confirmed the great benefit to arthritis of natural sunlight. In *Health and Light,* he proved with regard to his own arthritis that spending as much time as possible out of doors, walking or gardening, and receiving natural sunlight energy (even on dull days) directly thorugh the eyes, *minus sunglasses, spectacles, or contact lenses,* is highly beneficial in the control of this disease.

- The elimination from the diet of *vinegar, spices, tea, coffee,* and *alcohol*—especially sweet wines and liqueurs.

- *Calmness and emotional control.* Tension, fear, anger, hate, and so on do much to aggravate arthritis symptoms and increase suffering.

It must therefore be repeated again: *arthritis is a purely nutritional state and its logical treatment is a nutritional one.* Unfortunately, arthritis research foundations have been issuing statements for many years that nutritional therapy is totally without merit, thus discouraging most doctors from paying attention to their patients' diet. Any cure or improvement resulting from nutritional therapy has therefore been dismissed as a "spontaneous remission." There is now, however, too much solid evidence of sustained benefit from such therapy to justify this concept. Such a remission, of course, does occur.

Obesity
This is a far more serious condition than most people realize; it is now closely linked with diabetes, cholesterol-rich

gallstones, and coronary artery disease. Over 45 million Americans (twice the population of Canada) were overweight in 1978, and obesity among children is now reaching epidemic proportions.

It is generally believed that people become obese because they eat too much. Dr. Hay believed that obesity is far more often evidence of an imbalance in nutrition than the result of eating too much, and that its cause lies very frequently in the mixture of starches and proteins, or starches and acid fruits. He also strongly indicted refined carbohydrates, as did Cleave fifty years later.

The logical treatment for obesity, therefore, whether this is of slight or severe degree, is to correct the faulty eating habits that led to this condition. Compatible eating is especially effective. According to many reports I have received from Hay System followers, *merely avoiding warring mixtures is sufficient to reduce excess weight gradually — without even trying to do so; without feeling hungry; without wearisome calorie counting; and without resorting to crash diets, appetite suppressors, and dangerous drugs.* Dr. Hay warned that all so-called reducing remedies "should be avoided as you would the plague," because they are a snare and a delusion, and their very slight results are paid for at a fearful cost in vitality and health. His warning has now received ample confirmation in a report by the consumer magazine *Which?* of April 13, 1983; it had harsh words for certain fast weight loss products, which not only fail in their objective but also have unpleasant side effects.

Attempts to lose weight quickly are not recommended. Any change in the diet should be made gradually. To start losing weight, it is therefore sufficient just to become accustomed to separating the incompatible classes of foods into different meals. When this separation is well established, the number of alkaline-forming meals should be increased. An excellent and easy way of doing this (if desired) is to make breakfast consist solely of fruit, or fruit and yogurt, making the fruit one kind of fruit only. Doing so will cause no drop in energy for the day's work — *the energy for today is provided by the foods eaten yesterday;* eating a large breakfast actually ties up some energy during the morning. Dr. Hay always counseled that "the best breakfast of all is no breakfast at all"—but not if you are mixing incompatible foods.

Many people are not at all hungry for breakfast, but sheer habit forces them to eat. Dr. Hay always taught: *"Never eat anything of any kind at any time unless you feel really hungry. . . .* You will get far more nourishment out of foods that are eaten when you are very hungry than if these same foods are eaten without proper hunger."* This excellent rule is not only important for dieters but also for everyone who is health conscious. Cleave considered it so important that he listed it as rule number one in his "Natural Diet for Health" *(The Saccharine Disease,* page 188): *"Do not eat any food unless you definitely want it."* It is a fact that most of us eat far more food than we need. There is truth in the saying that "we live on a third of the food we eat—the doctor lives on the other two-thirds"!

There is no need to go without good, unprocessed, unrefined, whole food while dieting, provided that it is eaten compatibly. Even the so-called fattening foods—bread and potatoes—can be eaten with impunity, provided that the bread is whole wheat bread (preferably home-baked—see Part Four, "Recipes for Starch Meals"), the potatoes are cooked in their skins and the skins eaten, and care is taken not to "plaster" both the bread and potatoes with too much butter. Fats should be used with care by dieters, especially cream cheeses; cottage cheeses are best, as long as they contain no added salt. The intake of salt should be drastically reduced for dieters (and considerably reduced in the diet of most people).

Obesity is closely associated with constipation, indigestion, and arthritis. The advice that is good for the treatment of these conditions is therefore good for the treatment of obesity: removing the cause—refined carbohydrates, especially all sugars and *hidden* sugars, and incompatible food mixtures; ensuring that the bulk of the food intake consists of the alkaline-forming fresh vegetables, salads, and fruits; eliminating foods not recommended; eating as much food as possible in raw form; maintaining regularity; and not forgetting the daily ration of fresh, unprocessed bran, and other food supplements.

With regard to exercise—the time worn remedy for excessive deposits of fat—Dr. Hay warned that forced exercise should never be taken in order to lose weight: "Burning up the fats through exercise increases one's appetite tremendously, and consequently the total of foods of all kinds consumed." Exercise while losing weight should be of the moderate kind.

Paradoxically, compatible eating is equally helpful to people who are under weight! Both conditions are due to abnormal states of body chemistry. Therefore, just as compatible eating produces a steady loss of weight for those who are overweight, so will it also produce a gradual building up of weight for those who are too thin—the only difference being that thin people can make more use of the starch foods. Thin people should be warned, however, that they, too, will lose weight *at first*. This is no cause for concern and is merely an adjustment, "a throwing off of the old in preparation for the building of the new."

The Hay System is first and foremost a normalizing régime. This fact clearly indicates that nature works continually to restore us to the ideal in weight, stature, health, efficiency, and everything else, when we remove the obstacles in the way of her remarkable healing power.

Diabetes Mellitus (noninsulin-dependent type)
Of the two kinds, "late onset diabetes" and "early onset diabetes," Dr. Hay's writings concerned the former; the latter was rare in his time because children in the early 1900s did not consume fiber-deficient junk food as they do today.

About 2.5 percent of the US population (5.8 million people) are diagnosed diabetics and it is estimated that an additional 4 to 5 million have the symptoms but have not been diagnosed. For years their doctors have been advising them to cut down drastically on carbohydrate foods and eat a high fat diet. In November 1982, British doctors admitted that they had been on the wrong track and had been giving the wrong advice to their diabetic patients. *Dietary Recommendations for Diabetics for the 1980s — A Policy Statement by the British Diabetic Association (BDA)*, published in 1982, turned the conventional diet on its head, "because of its potential cardiovascular risks." Instead of the traditional low-carbohydrate, high-fat diet, this Policy Statement recommended a diet containing much less fat but *a high proportion of unrefined carbohydrate foods* — a remarkable tribute to the dietary concepts of Cleave, which, till the 1970s, were derided by his fellow physicians. The Policy Statement also recommends the avoidance of all sugar and emphasizes the value of fresh fruits and vegetables.

The BDA's new dietary recommendations provide striking confirmation and vindication of Dr. Hay's own beliefs and dietary recommendations at the beginning of the century; he, too, was convinced that he and his medical colleagues had been giving "the wrong advice"; he, too, advocated a diet containing a high proportion of unrefined "fibrous carbohydrate foods" instead of the traditional low-carbohydrate diet; and he, too, recommended strict moderation in fat intake and emphasized the value of plenty of fresh fruit and vegetables.

His dietary recommendations for diabetes, moreover, were enunciated, *seventy-one years before the publication of the BDA's Policy Statement in 1982*, in a paper read before the United States Warren County Medical Society in 1911. In this paper on diabetes mellitus, Dr. Hay stated:

> The very men and women whose daily food comes most nearly up to the standard of diet prescribed for diabetics are the men and women in whom the cases of diabetes are most numerous and most fatal. They are the people whose daily ration is filled with fish, flesh, and fowl, and in which but little room is left for bread and potatoes.

This paper is thought to be the very first piece of written material dealing with the Hay System. It was lost for nearly thirty years, but soon after Dr. Hay's death in 1940, it was fortunately found by the purchaser of his old desk, jammed along with other papers behind one of its drawers. It is of special value and significance for Dr. Hay's followers, it revealed that *he was having remarkable success in restoring former late onset diabetics to health, without drugs, eleven years before Banting and Best discovered insulin.* He did so by telling his patients "to quit the meat, eggs, and fish which had formed the principal part of their nourishment for so long and to eat a baked potato once a day, a slice of toasted whole wheat bread, and all the juicy fruits that were desired" (he had not at this stage developed the starch-protein concept). The improvement on this régime, he affirmed, "was marked and very gratifying to the patient, not only because of an increase in strength but in appetite and spirits, and what seemed at first strange, there never was a marked increase in the amount of sugar voided and this was even diminished. . . ." (He also instructed his patients to keep their bowel movements regular by every possible means, including daily two-quart enemas of cool, plain water.)

Dr. Hay's success in treating diabetics in this way convinced him completely that a strict adherence to his plan for long enough would result in a complete cure of all those cases in which there was no grave organic change. But to the medical pundits at that time, his treatment for diabetics was rank blasphemy. For one thing, diabetes had always been considered incurable; for another thing, all avenues of relief had been explored without success. *Yet here was a man who preached that diabetes was curable without the use of drugs.* They branded him a charlatan and ostracized him — they could do no less to safeguard their professional integrity.

Dr. Hay, dismissed as a "charlatan," was in truth an unrecognized and humble genius who had found the key, not only to diabetes mellitus, but to all the degenerative diseases.

Allergy

"Allergy," wrote Dr. Hay, "is a specific lack of body resistance to certain irritants, whether food, pollens, foreign proteins, or whatever," but, he affirmed, *the cause lies in the individual and not in the environment.*" The irritants are merely the secondary cause (irritants, here, meaning naturally occurring ones, not man-created environmental poisons in food, air, and water, to which the healthiest body has little resistance), the primary cause being almost wholly in what we eat and how we eat it, and in a state of disturbed body chemistry. He promised that a hay fever sufferer can so change his body chemistry "that he can bury his face in his former *bête noir*, no matter what this happens to be, without a single sneeze."

During the past few decades, very strong support for Dr. Hay's concept that allergies are linked to disturbed body chemistry has come to light through the work of Ott. In his book, *My Ivory Cellar*, he described a project to determine the action of ragweed pollen grains. While working on this project, he produced visible evidence that the primary cause of hay fever may be disturbed body chemistry and not the contact with the pollen grain as universally believed. Time-lapse microscopic photography revealed that grains of ragweed pollen placed in nasal secretion from hay fever sufferers immediately started to emit tiny droplets of liquid. These droplets did not form, however, when ragweed pollen grains were placed in nasal secretions from persons not subject to hay fever.

Ott surmised from this that the body chemistry of hay fever sufferers was exactly right to make the ragweed pollen grains give off the droplets of fluid, and that these could possibly be the factor that irritated the nasal membranes and not the mere contact with the outer surface of the pollen grains themselves. He suggested that if this is so, hay fever could then be prevented by altering the patient's chemical balance instead of trying merely to alleviate the trouble with medicines after the hay fever has once set in.

Compatible eating acts as a double protection against allergy:

as well as greatly improving the chemical balance (it takes about five years of correct eating to achieve—or approximate—the ideal state), it also ensures against the allergy-causing potential of incompletely digested proteins (see Chapter 2, "The Hay System Explained").

It is well known that, when proteins are incompletely broken down and imperfectly digested, they split into intermediate or large protein molecules that are actually toxic, instead of into amino acids, their proper end-products. Some of these protein molecules constitute the substance known as histamine, well-known to medical specialists as a toxic protein, which can be responsible for many common allergies such as hay fever, asthma, migraine, eczema, and urticaria. The liver of a healthy person can quickly destroy histamine, whereas a damaged liver cannot.

Munro relates, in *Man Alive, You're Half Dead!*, how he found an excellent way of testing his allergic patients for the toxic proteins created by the mixed meal. He used on them the histamine-destroying substance histaminase, and by doing so was able to discover "with a considerable degree of accuracy" to what extent the mixed meal produces toxic end-products. He found that these patients required more units of histaminase to control their symptoms when eating mixed meals than when eating correctly combined ones—proof that the mixed meal produces more histamine. Munro considered that this evidence alone was sufficient to justify compatible food combinations. When his patients were taught to avoid bad combinations, many lost their symptoms entirely. (Because one of the many benefits of natural yogurt—not the sugared and flavored kind—is its ability to inhibit the production of histamine, allergy sufferers might experience some relief from symptoms by eating this natural antihistamine daily—so much safer than the toxic drug form.)

A report of an allergy conference in *Hospital Doctor* of August 6, 1981, revealed that the management of the allergic patient in Britain at that time was worse than for almost any other disease. The usual treatment was suppression of the allergy symptoms by means of drugs and aerosols — treatment that deals only with the *manifestation* of the cause and not the fundamental cause itself: the patient's eating habits and (increasingly) chemical pollutants in his environment. Pioneers in the new discipline of clinical ecology, like Mackarness, who are tackling the fundamental causes of allergy, are having spectacular results, especially in cases where suspect food additives have been producing hyperactivity and serious behavioral problems in children. Needless to say, the concepts of these researchers in clinical ecology are challenging orthodox medical thinking and arousing the same medical disbelief and rejection as did the nutritional concepts of Dr. Hay.

The results of these pioneers, however, would be even more spectacular if they taught their patients how to improve their body chemistry by adopting compatible eating; these patients would then be able, within two or three months, to restore to their diet all the healthful natural foods to which they were formerly allergic, and as Dr. Hay promised, they would soon be able to bury their faces in their former *bête noir*, whether it be pollen, house dust, animal fur, synthetics, or whatever, "without a single sneeze."

It was encouraging to find, while doing research for this book, that in the 1930s at least one doctor in Britain agreed with Dr. Hay that warring mixtures are detrimental to allergy sufferers. In *The Treatment of Asthma* Dr. Harrington warns that mixtures of acid fruits, such as grapefruit, and starches should be avoided at the same meal, and that acid fruits taken with large quantities of bread and butter are especially bad for asthma sufferers.

Skin Diseases
Being visible, skin diseases are a valuable indication of the state of health of the whole body. Their cause, as with all other diseases, is traceable to a toxic state of the body. The disease itself is evidence of the body throwing off toxic debris by passing it through the skin.

Why, in some people, should it be passed through the

skin? The answer is that toxic debris finds an outlet through many different manifestations of the degenerative diseases, the particular form taken being determined by the specific resistance of the various organs. "Here," wrote Dr. Hay, "is where heredity comes in. The *form* of disease is determined largely by the inheritance, but the *fact* of disease is determined by the individual." It is therefore the weakest link in the hereditary chain that determines the organ, tissue, or function to give way first.

After nearly thirty years of applying the principles of natural treatment of disease, Dr. Hay affirmed that he had seen no case of psoriasis or eczema that did not disappear after a few weeks or a very few months of separation of the incompatible foods, even though both conditions failed to improve under the most scientific treatment of many prominent skin specialists. And he urged, "Treat all skin eruptions as external evidences of internal intoxication. Set about correcting all the causes of intoxication at once, and watch the results." These results, being on the outside of the body, can provide an excellent visible demonstration of the Hay System at work, and of its astonishing efficacy when faithfully carried out.

Much of this internal toxic state—Dr. Hay bluntly referred to it as "internal filth"—arises from the fermentation and putrefaction of incompletely digested carbohydrates. Once again, the troublemakers are sugar and white flour foods— but especially sugar where skin diseases are concerned. In *The Saccharine Disease,* Cleave confirms this fact: "The relationship of many cases of eczema, especially in children, to the consumption of sugar, sweets, and confectionary is well known, and in the author's opinion, chronic furunculosis is the surest sign of high sugar consumption *and is most quickly arrested by stopping it.*"

Some years ago, I witnessed a remarkable demonstration of this fact in the case of a ten-year-old boy who had had eczema since birth. He had been to specialist after specialist but was getting worse instead of better. At the age of ten, his eczema was so bad that his classmates shunned any contact with him, and his family was kept awake at night with his moanings and scratchings. When his mother, in despair, brought him to see me, his arms and legs were a solid weeping mass of eruptions. I instructed her to cut out all his sugary breakfast cereals, his colas and fizzy "pop" drinks, candy, cakes, and cookies, and to substitute fresh fruit for desserts at his main meal. I also instructed his mother how to make her own "no-kneading," whole wheat bread. Ten days later, she phoned to tell me that *the eczema had vanished,* that nothing remained but shadows where the weeping eruptions had been. I was totally astonished at the speed of this boy's recovery—*in ten days after ten years of misery and the total failure of medical treatment!* His mother said her son had been most cooperative, was enjoying his new diet—especially the home-baked bread!—and was thrilled to have normal healthy skin for the first time in his life. Significantly, no skin specialist consulted had ever mentioned "diet."

The first thing to do in the treatment of eczema and other skin diseases, therefore, is to eliminate all sugar and sugar-containing foods from the diet; the sugar acts by providing the right condition in the intestine to favor the proliferation of harmful products. When these are absorbed into the bloodstream, they can be responsible for acne, chronic boils, eczema, and many other skin conditions.

The second thing to do is to restore the body, as far as possible, to the proper chemical balance by adopting compatible eating.

Last, beauty-conscious women will be delighted to know that compatible eating does more than cure skin diseases; it also ensures a beautiful and flawless complexion. In *The Joy of Beauty*, Leslie Kenton affirms that the vital acid-alkaline balance is an important aspect of any diet for "super" health and beauty and one that most nutritional systems completely overlook. "For we can reach truly positive health—health beyond the simple absence of disease—and remain permanently healthy only when the foods we eat supply us with a surplus of alkaline-reacting foods."

The Common Cold

"Colds are not caught; they are created with the feet under the dinner table, and in no other way." This was Dr. Hay's common-sense belief.

The common belief, however, is that colds are created through germs—it is so much easier to look for the cause in a germ than in our wrong living habits. But the *primary* cause of colds is not the cold germ but the state of the body chemistry that provides a suitable soil for the proliferation of this type of germ. Moreover, if the cold germ were the primary cause of the common cold, then everybody, every-where, would have colds all the time. This is not the case, however, despite the fact that the germs found in the ex-cretions from the nose and throat during colds are the same, ubiquitous germs found anywhere at any time.

It is therefore evident that something protects the ones who escape infection, and this is the very thing that deter-mines the cause of colds. As Dr. Hay pointed out, "In-dividual susceptibility or immunity is determined by each individual's condition at the time, and if you are cultivat-ing an internal condition that makes for susceptibility then you may look for frequent colds when these are epidemic, or you can look for complete immunity during even the ex-treme peak of epidemic colds or influenza." Hay System adherents have proved the truth of this statement and found themselves virtually immune to colds, as I myself have done—my record being twenty years without so much as a sniffle.

Although much time-and-money-consuming research during the past fifty years has been directed at finding the causes and cure of the common cold, medical science ad-mits that these are still a mystery. Knowing the causes, Dr. Hay understandably questioned "what particular brand of stupidity could ever have made such research seemingly necessary in the first place?" He warned that no progress would ever be made until "the germ theory" was dropped and the fact accepted that *every cold is merely an expression of the body's effort to clean house.* If the cold is evidence of the body's effort to get rid of objectionable waste material that is hampering its normal functioning, then its prevention lies in the elimination of this hampering waste. But the usual treatment is not directed towards this elimination but to fussing with end results, to soothing the mucous membranes involved with sedative or antiseptic inhalants, cough remedies, and gargles. These remedies are directed towards *symptoms*, and not one is directed toward the removal of *the causes* that alone can produce the disagreeable and sometimes dangerous symptoms that we call a cold.

Nature herself indicates how to remove the causes by the fevers and loss of appetite that often accompany a severe cold. Therefore, the best possible thing to do is to cut out all meals and do a fruit juice fast or, preferably, a fruit fast. The saying "feed a cold and starve a fever" is badly misinterpreted. It really means that if you feed a cold, you will end up having to starve a fever. The fruit fast is very pleasant; as much of any one kind of fruit desired every two hours throughout the day, for several days or even a week. Each day a different fruit can be chosen.

There is, however, a speedy way of breaking up a cold, but it involves much self-discipline and should not be undertaken unless with the approval and advice of the family doctor or a qualified naturopath. It involves taking a hot bath at night, as hot as one can stand; sipping a quart of hot water and lemon juice while in the bath; staying in the bath till sweating freely; then wrapping up in a blanket and lying under heavy covers to continue the sweat as long as possible; taking a laxative in the morning on an empty stomach and eating no food till late afternoon, the first meal then consisting of fruit and vegetables, before returning to a normal régime. An effective but somewhat drastic remedy for a cold!

It is far better to live so that colds cannot develop; the day is fast approaching when we will be as ashamed to admit to a cold as to a term in prison. "But if you have sinned and a cold is the penalty," wrote Dr. Hay, "clean house just as nature would do through a longer time, but do it first!"

Headaches

A headache is one of the commonest afflictions that plague us, especially women.

It is generally believed that not much can be done for headaches, and heredity usually gets the blame, particularly if mother and grandmother have both been sufferers. Like every other disease, heredity largely determines the form, as specific resistances are inherited, but as Dr. Hay has pointed out over and over again, "Like disease of every other sort, headaches cannot be inherited but must be created by the individual."

Apart from those headaches caused by sunstroke or pressure on cervical nerves by displacement of the vertebrae, every case of headache marks a toxic state. In the case of migraine, for instance, each attack marks the end point of the body's toleration for the toxins that have caused the trouble. A migraine attack is nature's effort to unload these toxins so that the body can be restored to a less toxic state and its function improved to normal; hence the sickness, the vomiting (frequently), and loss of appetite. Most migraine sufferers report feeling better for a time after each attack. This improved state would continue for the sufferer, and there would be no more migraines if the causes were not repeated. But the causes *are* repeated, and the whole vicious circle starts again.

One of Dr. Hay's hundreds of successful cases is worth relating, this one being a pure case of serendipity. A woman of eighty-three asked to see him before a lecture in a college town because she had something very interesting to tell him. Her son had consulted Dr. Hay three months before for indigestion, and had been directed to combine his foods compatibly. She thought she would make it easier for her son to keep to his new regimen if she followed it also. To her immense astonishment, *within the first week* of doing so, she lost a continuous and often severe headache that had plagued her every day of her life since she was fifteen years old—*that is, for sixty-eight years!* and she had made no other change in her eating habits apart from combining her foods compatibly.

As well as eating compatibly, however, Dr. Hay advised "bringing the colon up to date and keeping it up to date" by means of thorough enemas, "for it is in the colon that so much starchy fermentation occurs due to the delay in discharging the unsplit starches found there." An enema alone, he affirmed, would cure a very large percentage of headaches. But in order to complete the guarantee of permanent relief, it was necessary to separate foods into compatible groups. "Any headache that persists in spite of this could be safely set down to pressure on the cranial nerves as they emit from the neck and can be taken care of perfectly by the osteopath or the chiropractor."

Headache is really a very simple thing to understand and to treat when considered from the standpoint of the cause — a toxic state of the body. When this self-created cause has been removed, the body itself makes the cure.

Dental Decay
To Dr. Hay toothache was merely an evidence of wrong chemical conditions of the body.

He affirmed that accumulation of the acid end-products of digestion and metabolism, or deficiencies in the normal alkaline reserve, is the entire cause not only of dental decay but also of all forms of inflammation of the gums and the entire category of mouth diseases.

No amount of cleanliness or meticulous hygiene of the mouth, he wrote, would have any effect on these disagreeable conditions if the food lacked the necessary elements for any length of time. The first evidences of trouble are red, marginal gums that later shrink and recede; the furred, fissured, or indented tongue, or the enlarged "papillae" so commonly seen on the tip of the average tongue; the early decay of the teeth; and crowding of the arch with the teeth out of line, interfering with the bite. Dr. Hay insisted that before any dentist is allowed to practice, his teachers should assure themselves that he knows the meaning of these evidences and how to meet the conditions.

The dentists, however, have paid almost no attention to wrong diet as a cause of these conditions. Since the end of the last century, they have been wholly concerned with the so-called "acid theory," which states that cavities are caused by "bacteria in acid fermentation" (bacteria producing corrosive acid by fermenting sugar and other refined carbohydrates) — the so-called "plaque." The acid theory has therefore focused research on attacks on the teeth from *without* and obscured the increasingly accepted fact that decay *primarily* starts from *within*, in the dentine below the enamel. This theory accounts for the truth that, despite their brilliant advances in dental technology, dentists are still no nearer to solving the problem of dental decay. It also accounts for the dental profession's naively eager acceptance of the fluoridation of water supplies as "a key measure" toward solving the problem, and for mistakenly dignifying it as "preventive medicine."

Such acceptance reveals a lamentable sweeping-aside of the fundamental cause of dental decay — the enormous present-day consumption of sugar, candy and other sugary carbohydrates. It also reveals a total ignorance of what preventive medicine is all about. In promoting this nostrum for dental decay, dentists are merely treating *the symptom* — cavities — instead of grappling with the *cause* — faulty nutrition. As Dr. Carstairs pointed out in a BBC Reith Lecture: "To allay the symptom while failing to explore and, if possible, eradicate the cause has always been bad medicine."

Dr. Hay would have called fluoridation an outstanding example of "bad medicine"; he continually emphasized the foolishness of trying to cure any condition without first removing the cause.

The dentists know very well that sugar is the chief cause of dental decay, but *always and only as it affects the teeth from without*. Thus they continually overlook the fact — well known to Dr. Hay sixty years ago, and revealed by recent medical findings — *that sugar not only wreaks havoc on the teeth but also on the body as a whole*, and is now known to be responsible for many of the crippling degenerative diseases such as those discussed in this chaper, and of the presently fatal degenerative diseases, coronary heart disease and cancer of the colon.

In *The Lancet* of February 5, 1983 (page 282, "Sugars and Dental Decay"), Dr. Aubrey Sheiham, of the Department of Community Health at The London Hospital Medical School states unequivocally: "Sugar is the principal cause of the most common disease in industrialized countries." He gives some excellent advice on how sugar intake should be reduced, but always in the context of its direct action on the tooth surfaces. Nowhere does he point out sugar's close link with the degenerative diseases, or recommend a diet that would ensure *resistance to cavity attacks from within the tooth.* But he does state that dental decay is preventable and that "enough is known about its prevention to mount a successful attack upon it."

No successful attack has yet been mounted. Dental advice about sugar reduction is generally "perfunctory," frequently soft-pedaled, and even promotes the belief that general nutrition *has nothing to do with making teeth more resistant to decay*—as in the Health Education Council's policy document *The Scientific Basis of Dental Health Education.*

One dentist and his wife, Richard and Elizabeth Cook, wholeheartedly disagree with this outrageous belief. In their book *Sugar Off!,* they outline an excellent do-it-yourself nutritional method of maintaining one's own dental health which virtually eliminates all sugars and sugar-containing foods and drinks. (Although they do occasionally resort to sugar substitutes.) Having come to the conclusion that dental health is too valuable to be left in the exclusive control of dentists, who are "trained to mend and pull teeth, not to advise on dietetics," this husband and wife team decided to go it alone with this book; they firmly believed that "no dentist can bestow or dispense dental health. This you have to get for yourself,"—*advice completely in line with Dr. Hay's concepts.*

Even more in line with Dr. Hay's somewhat revolutionary concepts, however, was the advice being propounded by dentist Dr. Martha Jones in the 1930s. According to a report of her work in *The New York Sun* of December 5, 1934, *"the gist of her theory is that good teeth depend on the degree of alkalinity in the diet, that unless the diet contains more alkalines than acids, decay is likely to occur."* For every serving of meat, eggs, or bread (all of which are acid-forming in their end-products), Jones advised two servings of fruits and vegetables. She said that root vegetables, such as turnips and sweet potatoes, leafy vegetables and fruits make an alkaline diet, with leafy vegetables—the thinner and greener the leaf the better—the most alkaline. Jones also taught that the diets of expectant mothers are essential to the development of their babies' teeth, and that the child's teeth will be strong and healthy *if the mother has a very alkaline diet.*

According to *Dental Products Report,* April 1975, *"dietary control* of cavities and gum disease may soon replace the tooth brush and dental floss as the mainstay of a healthy mouth." At the 110th midwinter meeting of the Chicago Dental Society, Dr. H.A. Huggins of Colorado Springs reported that tailoring diets to the needs of individual patients had produced remarkably good results, where brushing and flossing had failed. Moreover, blood sample studies from more than 7,000 people and trace mineral analysis of their hair had led to the conclusion that *dental disease is actually a whole body disease.* This conclusion is totally in accord with that of Dr. Hay and of Cleave, with regard to dental disease.

It appears, from the following remarkable case history described by Dr. Hay, that a correct diet can not only *prevent* dental decay but also *regenerate* cavities. He told how a young man had suffered from a row of cavities at the gum level that nearly encircled his upper and lower teeth. These were so sensitive to hot and cold, and sweet and sour, that he was living largely on cooked cereal; his dentist had insisted that it was useless to do anything for his cavities. At this time, the young man came across the Hay System and determined to give it a try. After six months, he visited his dentist who perceived no change in his mouth. Six months later, however, he found his teeth were no longer sensitive and he was able again to chew hard foods with comfort. When his dentist next examined his teeth, he was so astounded at what he saw that he gathered a group of dentists to see this unusual case.

> Every cavity was replaced by small deposits of secondary dentine—nature's effort at repairs—a scar tissue exactly suited to repair of the tissues of the teeth. This secondary dentine was as hard as the original enamel, as his dentist proved on testing it with a drill. As a result, the young man kept all his teeth, and reported that he was happier and healthier than he had ever been in his life of well over forty years, never tiring, or running into depressed states, but always cheerful and optimistic.

As far as dental decay is concerned, orthodox treatment has been unable to prevent it. Fluoridation has failed—the recent world-wide decline in dental decay in children is not related to either naturally occurring or artificial fluoridation—and there is evidence *which has never been disproved* that the latter is causing harm, ranging from dental fluorosis in children (the first sign of poisoning from too much fluoride) to skeletal fluorosis in the elderly. Dr. Hay counseled: "Take care of the whole man and the teeth will take care of themselves, with or without a toothbrush."

Postscript
Lack of space prevents further discussion of degenerative diseases in the context of compatible eating. But those discussed above are sufficient to confirm Dr. Hay's contention (and that of Cleave) that all degenerative disease has the same cause, no matter what its myriad manifestations; that its fundamental cause is improper diet and its cure "lies in food always and only."

Unfortunately, there are a few degenerative diseases that do not respond to correct nutrition. One of these is "paralysis agitans." Wrote Dr. Hay:

This is the so-called Parkinson's disease, a degenerative change in the nerves, supposedly in the centers of the sympathetic flexi. The condition is incurable by any means so far, though many theories have been advanced and many remedies tried. It is a lamentable fact that when nerves of either sensation or motion begin to die, it is impossible to do anything constructive toward a cure.

(Toward amelioration, yes—new drugs have helped considerably.)

Cancer—the second highest cause of death among adults in the Western nations, now killing about one of every seven Americans and afflicting 30 percent of the US population in one form or another—is another condition for which virtually nothing has been done to "cure." In *The New Ecologist* of November/December 1978, in his article "The National Cancer Institute and the Fifty-year Cover Up," Peter Barry Chowka quoted the following statement of Dr. Hay which was published in *Cancer Journal* in 1927:

> Think back over the years of cancer research, of the millions spent, the time consumed, the pains expended . . . and where are we still today? Isn't it time to take stock of our basic concept to see if there isn't something radically wrong to account for the years of utter and complete failure to date? . . . Cancer has been consistently on the increase . . . . *Is it possible that the cause of cancer is our departure from natural foods?*

In this same article, Chowka explains how, fifty years ago, encouraging leads established a clear relationship between diet and cancer, but focus by cancer establishments on symptomatic treatment rather than on prevention had virtually covered up the real answer to prevention and cure of cancer, *"the return to a healthy diet."*

Now, at long last, this close relationship between diet and cancer is again being recognized—seventy years after Dr. Hay showed the way. There are now increasing medical reports that 30 or even 50 percent of all cancer cases are the result of "unhealthy lifestyles" and *improper diet. Hospital Doctor* of June 16, 1983, reported that at a meeting of the Imperial Cancer Research Fund in London on June 13, a change in lifestyle and diet was suggested by Sir Richard Doll as "the key to cancer cure": "Stop smoking, drink less alcohol, become slim, and eat more fiber and vegetables and less animal fat and fatty dairy products."

Dr. Hay said truly when he wrote:

> Verily, we are dunces when it comes to our treatment of our own bodies, for we are misinterpreting nature's plainest warnings and trying to avoid even seeing them, covering them up with the action of so-called remedies instead of removing the whole foolish condition.

The truth is that we have fed our animals far more intelligently than we have fed ourselves. The rancher has always recognized that when his animals are fed correctly, they remain well, and when fed incorrectly they get sick. It is worth noting, here, and particularly significant to the argument of this book, that even the canine species benefits from compatible eating! The famous vet, "Buster" Lloyd-Jones, warned dog owners in *Love on a Lead*, "Don't mix biscuits with meat or gravies. It can cause digestive disturbance."

It is very encouraging that we are at last using more intelligence to feed ourselves. Organized medicine is now recognizing the worth of nutritional and preventive methods of treatment — and even of "complementary medicine"! It is also very encouraging that, whereas a short time ago people refused to accept responsibility for their own health, today there is an insatiable demand for any kind of self-help health care that offers an alternative to drugs.

We therefore feel that at no time could "a new look at the Hay System" be more appropriate. People are ready to listen to the rationality and truthfulness of its precepts as never before. And the rewards are great; few people who have conscientiously investigated the principles of correct food combinations and correctly applied them to their eating habits have failed to experience tangible results in a very short time. Dr. Hay reported:

> Thousands have found the mode of life so superior to anything they have ever before experienced that few ever return to less scientific modes of living, but continue to make the eating of their daily foods a scientific study because they have found that this pays better dividends than anything they have before encountered."

He also reported that, while enthusiastic about their state of health, they nearly all admit being deeply impressed with their *freedom from fear of disease in the future*.

For all enthusiastic devotees of the Hay System, Dr. Hay has special words of advice that are worth repeating. He told them *not to say too much about it;* not to make the mistake in their enthusiasm of trying to convert friends or relatives; not to force "saving knowledge" on the unwilling; to help when help is desired; and by their own good health, efficiency and youthful appearance to be the most effective advocates—far better than reams of arguments—for the truths of right eating.

The distinguished actor, Sir John Mills, is just such an advocate. When asked in a press interview some years ago how he looked "so astoundingly good at seventy," and why he had "hardly put on a pound in thirty years," he replied: "I've followed the same diet for thirty years—the main rule is do not mix protein with starch."

Another famous film star, Evelyn Laye, was also a devotee of the Hay System. In the *Sunday Graphic* of August 23, 1936, she told how she adopted this way of eating when working in Hollywood, after becoming thoroughly upset because of a prolonged period of eating the wrong kinds of food:

> In a day I felt an improvement. In two weeks I was on tiptoe with health and vitality and felt more wide awake and energetic. I am certain that the reason for so many minor ailments in later life, such as indigestion, nerves, and those

fits of what our kinder friends term "temperament" can be laid at the door of wrong eating in earlier days.

It is an interesting fact of great importance and significance that it is not the body but the brain that shows the first evidence of improving nutrition, and often does so "in a day" as Evelyn Laye and many others have experienced. As Dr. Hay pointed out, clear thinking and right thinking both depend far more on eating the right foods in the right way than people dream of. There is no doubt whatsoever that our present-day nutrient-deficient, processed and junk foods are responsible to a considerable degree for the great increase in many of society's present ills: serious personality problems in young children; ugly "temperament" at home, office, and factory; depression-caused suicides; broken marriages; juvenile delinquency; mental illness; appalling muggings, and ever more violent crime. The psychological effects of food are powerful and far-reaching and this is only now beginning to be understood.

It is therefore encouraging that the disastrous, psychological effects of our late twentieth-century diet are at last being thoroughly investigated. In *The Times* of August 1, 1983, Barbara Griggs reported, in an article headlined *"Sugar's Bitter Harvest,"* that, in the past two or three years, researchers in America have been looking for possible links between the many polluting and nutrient-destroying factors in our diet and the growth of violent crime. *These researchers have found that sugar is "the arch-criminal of the piece."* Its overconsumption can result in the condition known as hypoglycemia, or low blood sugar, "in which messages from the brain controlling mood, motivation, and learning are perpetually disrupted." "The result," she wrote, "may be a sudden burst of temper, aggression, changes of mood, confusion, fatigue, and irritability . . . caffeine, alcohol, smoking, and exposure to allergens can all trigger this unbalancing of the body chemistry, but *nothing triggers it faster, or more predictably than sugar."*

Barbara Griggs pointed out—as I, too, have pointed out

many times elsewhere – that the rise in sugar consumption has exactly paralleled the rise in violent crime. Significantly, a study in America in 1980 "showed that a large percentage of juvenile delinquents tested were found to be eating more than 400 pounds of sugar a year in various forms." Predictably, Professor A.J. Vlitos, Director General of the World Sugar Research Organization, the lobby for the world sugar industry, dismissed any evidence against sugar as "flimsy"!

The new interest in the sugar/crime hypothesis is evident in the fact that "Nutrition and Mental Health" was the theme of the 1983 McCarrison Conference held at St. Hugh's College, Oxford on September 23-25, with the approval of the World Health Organization. One of the speakers, Dr. Michael Colgan, cited studies showing that criminal behavior can be caused by bad food and prevented and treated by good food. Another speaker, Dr. Alexander Schauss, clinical criminologist and author of *Diet, Crime and Delinquency*, urged that both commercial concerns and the government should work with academicians in order to assess the true impact of diet on deviancy, behavior, and learning.

In *Man the Unknown*, Nobel Prize-winner Dr. Alexis Carrel made two profound observations, which are highly relevant to the present argument, "There is no doubt that consciousness is affected by the quantity and quality of the food. . . . The possession of natural health would enormously increase the happiness of man." In the light of these observations, the Hay System offers an important and wholly beneficial dimension not only for avoiding degenerative disease, but for successful, healthy and happy living.

4.
ANIMAL FATS—FACT AND FICTION

The total fat consumption of Western man today is far too high for health, and the medical establishment is advising the public to reduce it. *The Hay System, properly carried out, automatically reduces the consumption of all fats.* Unfortunately, the public is being brainwashed by propaganda into believing that butter and other animal fats are conducive to heart disease and should be replaced by margarine and vegetable oils. We do not believe that animal fat is the villain of human nutrition and have used dairy products throughout the recipe sections in Parts Three and Four; we believe that natural, unprocessed, fresh foods are the basis of health, and so cannot on any account advocate the completely unnatural, highly processed spreads and oils now being manufactured and sold for human consumption.

Just how grossly processed these spreads and oils are is described by Ross Hume Hall, Professor of Biochemistry at McMaster University, Canada, in his thoroughly researched and well documented book *Food for Nought*.

Briefly, the seeds—soy bean, cottonseed, rapeseed, and corn—are first shattered to release the oil. This is done mechanically or with chemical solvents. The latter is the preferred method because it releases more of the oil from the seeds. The chemical solvent is boiled off, but traces of up to 100 parts per million remain in the oil. These have to be reduced to the "permitted" level—about 10 parts per million. Depending on the source, however, the oil may contain undesirable "free fatty acids." These have to be removed by treating the oil at 140°–160°F with a solution of lye (caustic soda!). When the soap that forms settles out, the oil is skimmed off. It is then bleached and subjected to a deodorizing process for about twelve hours. Finally, it is treated with an antioxidant to retard oxidation—*rancidity*. The antioxidant is usually "butylated hydroxyanisole." (Antioxidants, which are used to prevent rancidity in many products, are made from petroleum and are considered by some authorities to be possible cancer-inducers.)

In order to harden the oil into spreads, it has to be subjected to a process known as hydrogenation. For this the oil has to be mixed "with a fresh or previously used nickel catalyst and subjected to hydrogen gas in a pressure reactor." This process, however, leaves up to 50 parts per million of nickel catalyst in the product. These used to be left in the oil, but now a "scavenging" process is required to remove the nickel because traces of this catalyst have been found to make the product more susceptible to oxidation. "The refining process," warns Hall, "leaves the oil almost completely devitalized . . . . For example, lecithin has been expurged; this natural substance is associated with fatty materials in their natural state. It is an emulsifying agent, and aids in the digestion of fat."

Hall warns that physicians are promoting the eating of commercially processed vegetable fat in lieu of butter and other animal fats, "knowing nothing of what they recommend."

Quite apart from the massive *chemical* treatment, the *high heat treatment* of oils and spreads is alone sufficient to condemn them as nutritionally inadequate foods. According to Dr. Norman Walker in *Natural Weight Control*, "If the fats have been treated in excess of 120°F, they will fail to be adequately treated by the pancreatic digestive juices and will not be available for use by the liver . . . thus their constructive nutritional value is destroyed." Yet many people have complete faith in the "constructive nutritional value" of margarine. They little know that many margarines are made of just those highly saturated fats they think they are avoiding and that the added coloring may be both carcinogenic and allergenic, causing hyperactivity in their children.

The "Fat Hypothesis"

The concept of eating these highly processed spreads and oils as a prevention against heart disease became a widely embraced medical dogma in the early 1970s, but it imposed much needless worry and very real anxiety upon millions of people. It is evolutionarily, epidemiologically, biologically, and historically unwarrantable — *especially historically*. In the early part of this century, when margarine was little used, coronary disease was almost unknown. It was still a rare disease in the 1920s. From then on there was a steep rise in its incidence. According to a paper entitled "A General Practitioner's View," presented at the Butter Information Council Seminar in 1977 by W.W. Yellowlees, one of Scotland's foremost heart specialists, in 1924 there were no cases of CHD in the wards of his hospital; but by 1954, there were over 300. CHD is now occurring in increasingly younger men.

According to the Medical Correspondent of the *Sunday Telegraph* of March 20, 1983, fatal heart attacks among businessmen in their late twenties and early thirties have been reported by the worldwide medical emergency service Europ Assistance. This service — which guarantees on-the-spot medical aid for British subscribers traveling abroad — "handled 115 fatal heart cases in the twenty-eight to thirty-six age group in 1983, compared with eighty-two cases in 1981, and seventy-three in 1980."

The anti-animal-fat, low cholesterol diet that enjoyed such a cult in the 1970s is now largely in disrepute. Recent studies have so failed to vindicate the "fat hypothesis" that there is now a remarkable medical turnaround, especially in the US.

An impressive example of this change in medical thinking is revealed by Dr. George V. Mann in the *New England*

Journal of Medicine, on September 22, 1977. He asserts that "a generation of research on the diet-heart question has ended in disarray. . . . Foundations, scientists, and the media, both lay and scientific, have promoted low-fat, low-cholesterol, polyunsaturated diets, and yet the epidemic continues unabated, cholesteremia in the population is unchanged, and *clinicians are unconvinced of efficacy.*"

Another example of this turnaround is contained in a report in May 1980 from the National Academy of Science and the National Research Council of America (considered the supreme court of science), which is quoted in the *British Medical Journal* of August 16, 1980 as stating that prevention of coronary heart disease cannot be achieved by means of dietary or medical reduction of cholesterol, and recommending that these measures should now be abandoned! Diet-conscious Americans received a big shock. And the members of the Food and Nutrition Board that produced the report were severely castigated as if they were heretics *for making recommendations which were so out of line with federal government agencies.*

Yet another example has been provided by one of the original promoters of the low-fat, low-cholesterol hypothesis, Professor Jens Dedichen of Oslo. He has frankly admitted in *T. Norske Laegeforen* in 1976 that the Norwegian policy to reduce fat intake for the past twenty-five years—for which he was personally responsible—has produced *no fall in coronary mortality but rather a steady increase,* and this despite a five-fold increase in Norway in soybean oil consumption. He also admitted greatly regretting the anxiety created in the population by his policy and that during these twenty-five years, it had become increasingly clear "that we are on the wrong track." For this admission, needless to say, he was severely censured by his fellow scientists.

Dedichen's findings have been confirmed by numerous studies that failed to produce convincing evidence of the "fat hypothesis," and which, moreover, claimed that although high blood cholesterol is *associated with* coronary heart disease, it does not *cause* CHD.

The latest study, and by far the largest and most important one of all, was conducted in the US. It was called MR FIT (Multiple Risk Factor Intervention Trial), cost more than $100 million, covered ten years, and involved two groups of 6,000 men each. One group was told to stop smoking, reduce saturated fats, eat more polyunsaturates, and take a drug to reduce blood pressure. The other group, serving as the control, was given no specific advice. The results were reported in the *Journal of the American Medical Association* on September 24, 1982 and were of the highest significance: after seven years, there was no difference in mortality from heart disease between the two groups.

This result, and those of many similar studies, have convinced many medical people of the fallacy of the "fat hypothesis." But zealots still continue to promote it even, in some cases, to the point of fanatical absurdity. *World Medicine*, for instance, reported on June 27, 1981 that in the US, Coca-Cola was "being recommended for young Americans in order to avoid those dangerous saturates in milk"!

The Dangers of Low-Fat, Low-Cholesterol Diets
Clinical trials of these diets have not produced the benefits that were expected of them and have produced evidence of harm that was not expected of them. For instance:

- The *Medical News Tribune* reported on December 18, 1971 that there was an increase in the US of malignancy in people eating polyunsaturated fats (highly processed vegetable oils and spreads).

- In Australia, the *Medical Journal Australia* reported in 1974 that five patients who had all enthusiastically followed a diet-heart regimen, substituting polyunsaturated margarine for butter, and polyunsaturated oils for cooking, developed malignant melanomas (a form of cancer).

- In 1973, *New England Journal of Medicine* published reports linking low-fat and low-cholesterol diets with gallstone formation. According to Professor B. Borgström, an outstanding leader in fat biochemistry, "a diet rich in poly-unsaturated fats will increase the risk of gallstones."

- Yellowlees, in his paper "A General Practitioner's View," pointed out that a sharp rise in deaths from heart disease was reported in America between 1909 and 1961, during which time there was also a *sharp rise* in the consumption of unsaturated fats and oils.

- Recent findings have shown that too drastic a reduction of cholesterol "may lead to adverse changes in aging cells so that they may not withstand the assault of incipient non-heart ailments." So wrote Dr. Cedric Carne in the *Sunday Express* of February 13, 1983, adding that "it has recently been discovered that cholesterol may protect us from non-heart diseases"! He also wrote in the *Sunday Express* of February 10, 1974, that the belief that eating margarine and vegetable oils reduces cholesterol and prevents heart disease is *"the great medical myth of our time."*

Animal fat—in moderation—is not the villain of the modern-day diet after all!

Cholesterol Is Vital for Health

Hall has stated, "Cholesterol is a requirement of every living cell, and we cannot live without it. It is the building block of sex hormones." According to Nathan Pritikin in his book *The Pritikin Program for Diet and Exercise,* cholesterol also helps to make bile acids for digestion.

It is not *the amount* of cholesterol, however, that is important but the *disturbed equilibrium between cholesterol and lecithin.* The latter emulsifies fats, helping to prepare them for absorption. There is no harm in food containing natural cholesterol—for instance, egg yolks, though very rich in cholesterol, are also high in lecithin and, at the same time, rich in vitamins and minerals. Such is the present obsession in America with cholesterol that there is now a dietary cult that requires that the nutrient-rich egg yolk be thrown out and only the white retained for eating. As the egg white is a protein of doubtful use for the body, this is surely a case of throwing out the baby with the bath water! It is significant that in "Diet Lipids and Heart Disease – A Review of Nutritional Evidence," a paper published in *Diet and Heart Disease* (the report of a 1982 International Symposium), Germaine S. Brisson reported that diet studies have revealed that "adding two eggs daily to or withdrawing them from the diet had no effect at all on serum cholesterol levels."

Cholesterol and Vitamin C

In *Science* February 16, 1973, a very important study by Dr. Emil Ginter of the Institute of Human Nutrition in Bratislava, Czechoslovakia, revealed that vitamin C is an important link in the conversion of cholesterol into valuable bile acids, and that a *lack* of vitamin C can cause high serum cholesterol and promote the onset of atherosclerosis. According to Ginter's study, increasing vitamin C means more bile acids and this means that cholesterol remains in solution and does not precipitate out as gallstones or arterial "plaque."

In *The Lancet* December 11, 1971, research by pathologist Constance Spittle of Pindersfield Hospital, Wakefield, Yorkshire, also revealed the importance of vitamin C to cholesterol and bile acids. Her experiments to test the relationship of vitamin C intake to serum cholesterol levels produced very interesting results. In healthy people under twenty-five years of age, mean cholesterol levels dropped during a period of vitamin C therapy, but in atherosclerosis patients, vitamin C therapy led to a pronounced rise in cholesterol. Spittle believed this was due to "the mobilization of arterial cholesterol" – in other words, the life-threatening, hardened cholesterol in arterial plaque was loosened and washed out by the action of vitamin C. According to these results, vitamin C could be a specific therapy not only for *preventing* atherosclerosis but also for effectively treating it even where the disease is advanced.

Judging from the findings of both Ginter and Spittle, if

there is plenty of vitamin C in the diet—*such as in the high vegetable and fruit regimen recommended in this book*—the fats required by the body can be eaten and metabolized so that they cause neither gallstones, nor atherosclerosis, nor any other trouble.

Fat Is Vital for Health

The late Adelle Davis, an outstanding American nutritionist, has described how important fat is to health, especially for the proper functioning of the gall bladder.

In *Let's Eat Right to Keep Fit,* she wrote:

> A certain amount of fat is necessary to stimulate the production of bile and the fat-digesting enzyme, lipase. Only when fat enters the intestine, does the gall bladder empty itself vigorously. Without fat (i.e. *natural* fat) too little bile is formed and the gall bladder holds its reserve bile. This faulty emptying may be a factor contributing to the formation of gallstones.

Fat is also vital for the absorption of the fat soluble vitamins A, D, E, and K. Without the presence of fat and bile, these vitamins cannot be carried across the intestinal wall into the blood.

It must be repeated: naturally occurring fat is not the villain in the modern-day diet.

Refined Sugar Is the Villain

Since the early days of this century, nutritionally minded doctors, dentists, and scientists have given many warnings that refined sugar is damaging our health. But these warnings fell on deaf ears until the 1970s, when the research and writings of Cleave and his coworkers and converts produced evidence *as never before* that refined sugar and other refined carbohydrates, such as white bread and flour, were creating an epidemic of diseases that were wrecking the human body.

It is Cleave's revolutionary concept that most diseases that are plaguing modern man are just different manifestations of one master disease, which he terms "the saccharine disease" (saccharine being pronounced like the river Rhine, and having nothing to do with saccharin, the chemical sweetener). This concept has been hailed internationally as one of the most important medical discoveries of this century and has been responsible for an astonishing change in medical thinking regarding the importance in our diet of fiber-rich food such as whole wheat bread and bran.

The term "saccharine disease" refers to all those conditions that Cleave advances as due to the taking of sugar, either primarily as such, or secondarily via the digestion of starch in white flour and other refined carbohydrates. These conditions constitute a formidable list of sugar-linked diseases, *including coronary disease.* Significantly, the steep rise in CHD since the early part of this century has been concurrent with an enormous increase in sugar consumption. But there has not been a similar enormous increase in fat consumption, although there has been an appreciable increase in this also. This increase, it should be pointed out, has not been in butter and other animal fats but in the highly processed margarines and cooking oils arbitrarily ingested in so many present-day foods: potato chips, the ubiquitous french fries with everything, including those served at school, instant foods, pastries, cakes, ice cream (of which increasing *millions* of gallons are now consumed yearly), cookies, and so on.

The recent slight decrease in CHD deaths reported in the early 1980s has therefore been attributed to this increased consumption of processed fats. Since the 1960s, however, there has been a *marked decrease* in the consumption of sugar. There has also been a *marked increase* in the consumption of high-fiber whole wheat bread and bran. Thus, the *total* of refined carbohydrates has decreased in the last twenty years. *This is the factor most likely to be responsible for the recent reduction in CHD deaths, and not that of increased margarine and plant oil consumption.* This conclusion is in perfect agreement with Cleave's concepts.

In his book *The Saccharine Disease,* he puts forward irrefutable arguments and evidence, which make a nonsense of the "fat hypothesis." He reveals the fallacy of treating coronary disease as an isolated disease and stresses that it is one of a group of interrelated diseases, often occurring with others—diabetes and obesity, in particular—in the same patient. He is completely confident that "the key to causation of coronary thrombosis lies in the causation of diabetes (and also of obesity)." He is equally confident that the "absolutely dominant cause" of both diabetes and obesity lies in the overconsumption of refined carbohydrates, sugar especially, where the loss of fiber deceives the appetite and sense of satiety, and also causes an abnormally swift and massive absorption.

It is this clinical association with diabetes and obesity that so precisely indicts sugar, not fat, as the cause of heart disease. That fat is not the cause is confirmed by the freedom from coronary disease, which has been carefully observed in certain East African tribes—the Masai (reported in the *British Medical Journal* on July 31, 1971) and the Samburu (reported by A.G. Shafer et al in the *East African Medical Journal* in 1969)—despite diets containing enormous quantities of animal fat by our standards.

Fiber Is the Crux of the Argument

As the fiber content of the diet goes up, so the blood level of cholesterol goes down. According to Ross in *Food for Nought,* this has been confirmed by experiments in animals and humans, and H.C. Trowel concluded in the *American Journal of Clinical Nutrition* in 1972 that fiber-rich foods therefore constitute an important protective factor against coronary disease.

Regrettably, the obsession with cholesterol levels has blinded the "fat" protagonists to the importance of a nutritionally adequate, high-fiber, whole food diet. The whole focus of the "fat hypothesis" has been on preventing coronary disease merely by means of *fat modifications.*

More regrettably, this obsession has delayed the recognition that such a nutritionally adequate diet not only offers a simple do-it-yourself means of preventing coronary disease and its clinically associated diseases, but also of preventing the many other manifestations of "the saccharine disease."

Yellowlees, President of the nutritionally oriented McCarrison Society, scathingly summed up the complete absurdity of these "fat modifications" when he said while delivering the 1978 James McKenzie Lecture (published in the *Journal of the Royal College of General Practitioners* in January 1979):

> Obsession with cholesterol levels has led to some extraordinary dietary cults. These would have us substitute margarine for butter, restrict our egg consumption to three a week, and make the taking of cream a sin. (Whoever heard of anything so absurd as strawberries and skimmed milk?)

There is therefore no need to refrain from using dairy products in the recipes set out in Parts Three and Four of this book (unless for economy reasons or on doctor's orders), provided the refined carbohydrates are eschewed, and the diet contains enough fiber-rich and fresh "whole" foods.

5.
THE PROOF OF THE PUDDING . . .

The following case histories and extracts from letters provide evidence of many benefits experienced by adherents of compatible eating. We hope that readers new to the system will find them both helpful and encouraging.

Twenty-five years ago Cathy was sent to me by her doctor, who frankly admitted that the usual medical therapies could do nothing for her. She was so ill with asthma that she was on the point of giving up her job—her sole source of livelihood. A few weeks after adopting compatible meals, she felt so much better that she not only retained her job but took on a thrice weekly evening one as well. She has remained an enthusiastic adherent ever since, and has never looked back. Her doctor was delighted, and promptly sent me another patient!

Barbara had been ill off and on for nearly ten years—diarrhea (irritable colon); allergies to beef, cheese, milk, cream, tea, and coffee; palpitation (tachycardia) for which she was prescribed a heart drug that made her very ill. Treatment for eight years from an allergist failed to help very much. She deteriorated in health, was constantly tired both mentally and physically, and had no interest in living. In desperation, she commenced eating compatibly mixed foods and *within two days*, to her great surprise, she began to feel distinctly better. Within thirteen days, her bimonthly allergy skin tests were negative for the first time. Within sixteen days, she wrote to say that she not only felt better but also looked better than she had for many years. At the end of two months, she was able to eat most of the foods that had been causing trouble.

For eight years, Anna had been bedeviled with allergies to a number of foods, and with a skin disease related to the allergies. She consulted specialist after specialist but experienced no relief from her miseries. Within two months of adopting compatible eating, the skin disease cleared completely and she was able to eat virtually all the foods to which she had previously been allergic. Significantly, no specialist consulted had made any suggestions regarding her diet.

"As I was desperate to find a remedy for indigestion (which was waking me up almost every night) I decided to try — though without much hope of success — the Don't Mix Foods That Fight Diet. And now I have to confess — the results have been remarkable! Within two weeks, I lost six pounds (which had been creeping up on me as "middle-aged spread"!) without feeling the least bit hungry. The rheumaticky pains in my hands have improved, and neither my husband nor I have had a cold, despite our office being full of them all winter long. I am so very grateful for being enlightened into sounder health and digestion."

"At the age of five, I developed asthma, but eventually overcame it by the time I was forty, through reading health books and gaining knowledge of how bad white flour is. Since then, for the last eight years, I have had to fight an allergic reaction to food, which has resulted in a rash; as soon as I found out which food was the culprit another would take its place. The *first day* of "compatible eating" I noticed a great improvement in the reaction of my skin and I can now eat all the foods that I could not before, with no sign of a rash.

I am so delighted with the results. It is certainly not hard to keep to this regimen, when the outcome is good health."

"The food I am eating now has improved my health already, and I am sure it will continue to do so. I feel much fitter, *so soon* after starting to eat this way. Thank you again."

"It was following your advice twenty-four years ago that we cured our eldest son's constant coughs (at school three weeks, away from school three weeks, and so on) when specialists and doctors had failed and said he would probably grow out of it when he was twelve—he was then seven years old!"

"I am putting compatible eating into practice and already I am less stiff than usual with arthritis and have lost four pounds. This is in a few days. I am most grateful."

"There is no doubt in my mind that I am already benefiting from the diet. It is years since I felt so well and happy. In fact now, at sixty, I feel ten years younger than I did at fifty. . . . My rescue is like a miracle, and I thank God daily for it when I happily tackle my household chores or go for long, long country walks. It's good to be alive and well and enjoying it all."

"Three years ago I was seriously ill with aplastic anemia, because my bone marrow was not making the red blood corpuscles I needed. I had no energy, could not walk far or do much, and some of my friends thought I was going to die.

"Although my specialist gave me every care, she said *there was no cure in my case,* and I would need blood transfusions for the rest of my life. I had these in the hospital every five and half weeks, and the outlook seemed bleak.

"But I would not accept the fact that I was incurable. For some time, I had been searching for a healthy diet, particularly after reading *Your Daily Food.* So I went to a qualified naturopath, who put me on a diet that followed all your principles. Within three months, the time between transfusions gradually lengthened, until I lasted for eighteen weeks. Then I had my twelfth and last transfusion. Fifteen months after starting the diet, my bone marrow began to work again and my hemoglobin (red cell corpuscle count) gradually began to rise, and two years later is continuing to do so. I am so well that recently I was able to tour the Rockies in Canada, without fatigue. I am sure that the diet helped in my cure, and am eternally grateful."

Four months later this same correspondent wrote:

"I am sure you will be glad to know how very well I am. I have made excellent progress since writing to you in December. My blood count made a big jump, and the specialist says I may have reached the normal figure for a woman of my age (sixty-five years). Anyway, I feel marvelously well, and it's really quite amazing when I think how ill I was three years ago, when the specialist intimated that I had no hope of a cure."

"Way back in the summer, I gave your Don't Mix Foods That Fight regimen to one of our patients who was suffering so much from psoriasis—a wretched skin condition. I didn't think she had taken to the idea, but we had a letter this week (December 1982) to say that she had followed your advice and her skin was remarkably better! And so the good work goes on."

"My husband and I are completely 'sold' on your compatible eating. . . . As you said, it is a way of life, not a diet, and we feel so well and full of energy. We have lost the weight we needed to lose, and I really am now convinced about the importance of separating the carbs and proteins in the diet."

"My mother has triumphantly reported that after four weeks

of compatible eating, she has lost six pounds without even trying and without feeling hungry. She feels fitter than she has for years."

"Though I have been a food reformer and vegetarian for the last ten years or so, my health has never been very good and I was very unhappy about it because I wanted so much to tell people around me of the benefits of food reform. You have showed me my mistake—and I think the mistake of many others, especially those who give up meat—*an excess of starch*. For me it was bread, whole grain bread. As it was 'good for me,' I simply indulged in it, *every meal and between meals!* I felt more and more tired with no real 'joie de vivre.' The starch-protein theory is, I am convinced, absolutely exact, and digestion seems much easier after only a week of separating incompatible foods."

"We have been following the 'protein or starch only at one meal diet' now for some time and seem to derive considerable benefit from it. The results speak for themselves. My husband and I notice the difference very quickly between eating a 'normal' meal (protein and starch) and a compatibly combined one. After an occasional 'orthodox' meal—when our work schedule is very tight—we feel burpy, windy, and acidy in the throat and stomach, whereas after your suggested meal we feel fine."

"Since last November I have had such difficulty walking after sitting down for short periods. A few days (truly!) after starting to eat compatibly, I was able to move without pain. My friends were amazed, as indeed was I. My husband has been wonderful—joining me in the early weeks with the result that he has lost one and a half stones [twenty-one pounds], and I, too, am now 8 st. 5 lbs. [117 pounds] from 10 st. 6 lbs. [146 pounds]. It was so effortless. There was an amusing incident in Waitrose [a grocery store] recently when, waiting at the checkout, a lady commented on the food in my basket and said she wished she could eat food like that (oatmeal, honey, cream, rye bread, butter) but she had a weight problem and pointed wistfully to her purchases—Nimble bread, Outline margarine, low calorie soups and drinks, Marvel milk. I couldn't resist telling her about the Hay System. I am so thankful I started eating this way because without it I should still be ten and a half stone [147 pounds] (at least!) and experiencing discomfort in my knees. I can quite honestly say it has completely changed my outlook on life. I feel marvelous. Thank you."

The experiences related in these letters, and in countless others I have received over the past forty years, are convincing evidence of the innate power of the body to heal, strengthen, and restore. By removing many obstacles, in the way of this healing power, compatible eating releases the marvelous capacity of the body to renew itself and throw off disease. A new look at the Hay System is indeed long overdue.

PART TWO

THE HAY SYSTEM IN PRACTICE
by
Jean Joice

6.

HOW TO BEGIN

The joy of the Hay System is its flexibility; it is not a rigid diet to be endured but a delicious way of eating for health and well-being, which can be enjoyed indefinitely.

Although this section of the book includes menus and recipes to help new converts to get started, we hope that readers will adapt their own favorite recipes and find new and imaginative ways of serving the wide range of delicious natural foods that are available season by season. There are now many books containing imaginative ideas for preparing the fruits and vegetables that are such an important part of the Hay System, and some of these are listed in the "Further Reading" section at the end of the book.

The detailed chart of compatible foods on pages 127 and 128 will help you to assemble meals until this way of eating becomes second nature.

The rules of the Hay System, fully explained in Chapter 2, "The Hay System Explained," are very simple:

1. Starches and sugars should not be eaten with proteins and acid fruits at the same meal.
2. Vegetables, salads, and fruits should form the major part of the diet.
3. Proteins, starches, and fats should be eaten in small quantities.
4. Only whole grains and unprocessed starches should be

used, and all refined and processed foods should be eliminated from the diet. This particularly applies to white flour and sugar and all foods containing them, all highly processed fats such as margarine, and all highly colored and sweetened foods and drinks such as soft drinks.

5. An interval of four to four-and-a-half hours should elapse between meals of different character.

The easiest way to put these rules into practice and to achieve the ideal ratio of four to one between the valuable alkaline-forming foods (vegetables, salads, and fresh fruits) and the acid-forming foods (meat, fish, eggs, cheese, and grains) is to arrange the day's meals so that animal protein is eaten only once a day, cereal starches are eaten only once a day, and the third meal contains neither, but consists only of fruit with milk or yogurt. It is usually most convenient to take this essential alkaline meal at breakfast, but, if a starch breakfast is preferred, an alkaline meal consisting of salad, fruit, and yogurt could be taken either at midday or in the evening. A comprehensive list of alkaline-forming foods is included at the end of the book to help you select foods for this very important meal.

Another, perhaps unexpected, feature of the Hay System is that although it excludes all highly processed convenience foods, the time needed to prepare food is usually far less than for the conventional cooked, mixed meal. Meals are simpler and easier to prepare, containing, as they do a high proportion of raw fruits and vegetables with their health-giving enzymes, minerals, and vitamins intact. Dr. Hay emphasized that simple meals are far better for health because they are less taxing for the digestive system. The suggested menus are therefore usually for two-course meals, consisting of one main dish with salad or freshly cooked vegetables, followed by fresh fruit in season. The three-course meal consisting of an appetizer, a main course, and a dessert should be regarded as an occasional treat for weekends, holidays, or when entertaining. Those who give the system a

fair trial will be surprised to find how satisfying and delicious this new way of eating can be, and how sugary
"treats," once relished, are no longer wanted.

On the following pages are listed the foods recommended
for protein, carbohydrate, and alkaline meals, and a "black
list" of foods to be avoided. Unfortunately this list is longer
than when Dr. Hay was writing because of the tremendous
growth of food technology and the ever increasing number of synthetic additives used in food processing. It is not
only because of the many additives they contain that factory foods should be avoided, but because they no longer
retain their natural complement of fiber, vitamins, and
minerals *in their correct proportion to one another.* This is a most
important factor, which is often overlooked, for all natural
whole foods contain the micronutrients essential for their
complete metabolism.

If the "foods to avoid" list looks somewhat daunting, it
is best to concentrate on the many delicious foods that *are*
available in the recommended lists—many of these more
readily available now than for many years, thanks to an increasing awareness of the importance of the "wholeness"
principle in the growing and preparation of food.

Foods for a Protein Meal

Proteins

Meats of all kinds
Fish
Shellfish
Chicken
Game
Eggs
Cheese—the natural variety,
   not processed
Nuts*
Mushrooms
Seeds*
Milk***—fresh milk only,
   not homogenized
Yogurt

*Fats**

Butter
Cream
Egg yolks
Olive oil (cold pressed)
Sunflower seed oil (cold
   pressed)

Sugar Substitutes

Diluted frozen orange
   juice
Honey in strict moderation
Maple syrup in strict
   moderation
Raisins and raisin juice*

Vegetables*
All green vegetables
All root vegetables (but
  not potatoes)
Mushrooms
(Spinach and *cooked*
  tomatoes are best not
  eaten more than once a
  week because of their
  high acid content)

Fruits
Apples
Apricots
Bluberries
Cherries
Grapefruit
Grapes
Lemons
Mangoes
Nectarines
Pears
Peaches
Prunes (Santa Clara)
Raspberries
Strawberries
Tangerines

Salad ingredients
Avocados
Beets
Cabbage
Carrots
Celery
Chicory
Cucumber
Fennel root
Legumes – sprouted
Mustard greens and
  garden cress
Lettuce
Parsley
Green peppers
Red peppers
Radishes
Seeds – sprouted
Tomatoes
Watercress

Salad dressings
French dressing
Cream dressing
Mayonnaise (homemade)
Use lemon juice or apple
  cider vinegar

*Note: Raisins, nuts, seeds, fats, salad ingredients, and vegetables combine with all meals.

**Fats: All fats are used in very small quantities, and although cream is used in some recipes, it is almost always used *instead* of another, possibly more concentrated, fat such as butter. If properly applied, the Hay System is a low-fat way of eating and automatically eliminates "hidden fats."

***Milk should be used sparingly by adults. It is intended by nature for young mammals! For adults it can be a great mucus-former. It combines best with fruits and vegetables, and salads, but can be used in small quantities with starches and proteins.

Foods for a Starch Meal

Cereals and grains
Whole grains: wheat; oats; barley; rice (brown, unpolished); rye; corn; millet; buckwheat

Bread made from 100% whole-grain flour
Flour—100% and 85% whole-grain

Sweet Fruits
(All fresh fruits should be completely ripe)
Bananas
Dates
Figs (fresh or dried)
Grapes (only very sweet varieties)
Papayas (very ripe)
Pears (very sweet varieties)
Raisins

Vegetables
All green vegetables
All root vegetables
Potatoes (cooked in their skins and the skins eaten)
Mushrooms

Milk
Use in *moderate* amounts only

Sugars
Honey
Molasses
Maple syrup (not synthetic)
Brown sugar
(All sugars should be used in strict moderation. Avoid "hidden" sugars such as those in commerical flavored yogurt, bottled fruit drinks, and so on.)

Eggs
Yolks only, but "compromise" occasionally and use whole eggs

Fats
(As for a protein meal)
Butter
Cream
Egg yolks
Olive oil (cold pressed)
Sunflower seed oil (cold pressed)

Salad dressings
Sweet or sour cream
Olive oil (cold pressed)
Mashed uncooked tomato mixed with oil, paprika, and seasoning

Unprocessed wheat germ and unprocessed bran should be taken daily

Foods for an Alkaline Meal
Acid fruits, milk, or yogurt as listed for a protein meal. All green and root vegetables; all salad vegetables; fats as for a protein meal; seeds such as sunflower seeds, almonds, sprouted seeds, and legumes.

A starch version of the alkaline meal can consist of potatoes, cooked in their skins and the skins eaten, served with butter and accompanied by a salad or cooked green vegetables. For this meal any fruit to finish should be selected from the list for starch meals.

Drinks
It is best not to drink at all with meals. The rule should always be: drink only when thirsty. However, if it is difficult to go without, the following suggestions may help.

With a protein meal
Weak tea or coffee (not instant) but no cereal coffee substitutes. Ceylon tea that is low in tannin or maté tea are preferable to very strong teas. Herb teas are excellent. All teas should be taken without sugar.

Fruit juices made from fresh acid fruits preferably diluted with a little spring water. Apple juice with Perrier water makes a good thirst quencher in hot weather.

Do not drink milk with a meat meal. Milk should be regarded as a food not a drink and taken only in moderation.

With a starch meal
Tea, coffee, or herb teas as above, and cereal coffee substitutes may be taken.

Fresh tomato juice and raw vegetable juices but not acid fruit juices. However, very sweet grape juice is permissible.

With an alkaline meal
As for a protein meal. However, because milk combines best with fruits and vegetables, it may be taken with a fruit breakfast.

Foods to Avoid

All refined carbohydrates. This means sugar in all forms, particularly white sugar, and all food and drinks containing it.

It also means white flour and all foods made with it such as bread, cakes, cookies, pastry, and dessert; also white polished rice and other refined grains such as tapioca.

Avoid carbonated and fruit-flavored soft drinks, and all bottled fruit drinks — even the so-called health soft drinks because these contain an appreciable amount of sugar. Watch out in particular for "hidden" sugars.

Read all food labels carefully, because sugar is contained in more foods than you might expect. Most muesli cereals, promoted as "health foods," contain up to 26 percent sugar. The "high fiber" cereals are also high in sugar; most commercial ice cream contains over 20 percent; tomato ketchup, over 20 percent; and salad dressing, 18 percent. Some sweet pickles contain over 30 percent sugar; most fruit yogurts, over 10 percent; and cola drinks, 10 percent. Even the relatively innocent baked beans, containing no other additives, have a sugar content of 5 percent, and often the zweiback on which babies cut their teeth contains up to 30 percent sugar. Many toothpastes also contain sugar.

Most processed and instant foods should be avoided because of the additives they contain. These are colorings, preservatives, flavor enhancers, emulsifiers and stabilizers, added by food manufacturers to "improve" appearance and flavor, and to prolong shelf life. Although new synthetic additives undergo rigorous tests, no one really knows what their long term effects on the human body may be, or the synergistic effect of an ever increasing number. Many are under attack as the cause of hyperactivity in children. Highly colored foods are particularly dangerous in this respect.

The eight largest groups of additives are flavors and flavor enhancers such as monosodium glutamate; thickeners and stabilizers; emulsifiers; food acids; colors; preservatives; antioxidants; and sweeteners. The only safe rule is to read all food labels and avoid any product containing any of these additives. Butylated hydroxyanisole (BHT) in particular has been banned in many countries after tests indicated that it could lead to liver and kidney damage and increases in blood fat and cholesterol.

For a detailed and explicit account of the additives used in processed foods, it is well worth reading *The Right Way to Eat* by Miriam Polunin; other foods to avoid because of additives are dried fruit preserved with sulphur dioxide; and prepared meats, including bacon, containing sodium nitrate and sodium nitrite, which in certain conditions can be cancer inducing.

Virtually all canned foods should be avoided; battery eggs and chickens; pickles; legumes (unless sprouted); cranberries; and rhubarb and plums (because of a high acid content). The use of salt should be reduced as much as possible and all heavily salted foods, such as salted peanuts, avoided altogether.

Fried foods should be omitted except for very occasional use. Instant coffee should never be used; tea or freshly ground filtered coffee may be used in moderation.

Basic Essentials for the Hay System Larder

Fruit, vegetables, and salad ingredients
It makes good sense to buy only what you need for a short time ahead, especially where fresh fruit and vegetables are concerned. If possible, buy organically grown vegetables or grow your own. Fresh foods start to deteriorate from the moment they are picked, so buy the freshest you can find and store them in the refrigerator, if there is room, or in a cool place until needed. All fruits and vegetables, especially from nonorganic sources, should be thoroughly washed. In the case of apples, pears, and so on, it is best to peel them.

Grains and stoneground wholewheat flours
Keep them in a cool place and use them within three months or less. Whole grains and flours that contain the germ will

not keep indefinitely and should always be used as soon as possible. The same thing applies to brown rice and whole-grain pasta, such as macaroni and spaghetti, and to seeds and nuts, particularly shelled nuts, even when vacuum packed.

Fresh wheat germ
This particularly valuable food supplement contains the vitamin B-complex, vitamin E, and EFA (essential fatty acids). Buy wheat germ only from a supplier who has a fast turnover, and store it in the refrigerator because it can go rancid very quickly. It can be sprinkled on cereals or used as a substitute for breadcrumbs in cooking.

Bran
This is another excellent addition to the diet, though if real whole wheat bread and plenty of vegetables are eaten, there should be enough fiber in the diet to solve any constipation problems, without additional bran. However, apart from supplying fiber, bran is also an excellent source of vitamin B_1, calcium, and iron. It, too, should be stored in the refrigerator.

Steel cut oatmeal (medium)
This is useful for making quick and delicious cooked cereal and for making oatcakes. It is cheaper than packaged cereals and far more nutritious. Oats can be used as a foundation for a homemade muesli.

Dried yeast
Use this for making bread. It keeps fairly well and is a good alternative to fresh yeast if it is difficult to obtain.

Fats and oils
Use only fresh, unsalted, or slightly salted butter and cold pressed sunflower seed oil or good olive oil of first extraction.
   The consumption of all fats should be decreased, and food

should not be fried. The digestibility of a fat depends on its being heated as little as possible during processing. (All margarines are highly processed—see Chapter 4). Fresh butter and vegetable oils contain the important EFA factor, and the fat soluble vitamins A, D, and E, whose absorption depends on EFA. Butter and oils of first extraction have the highest content of vitamins A and E. Again, buy only what you need for immediate use and store it in the refrigerator. Fresh butter can also be stored very successfully in the freezer.

Sea salt

It contains valuable trace elements but should be used very sparingly. Most of us consume too much salt and should cut down on its use as much as possible. The use of dried or fresh herbs for seasoning can help considerably to reduce the need for salt.

Honey

Provided it is organically produced and not blended with sugar, honey can be used occasionally as a sweetener.

Cider vinegar

Only cider vinegar should be used for salad dressings. Malt vinegar should never be used.

Dried fruits

These can be very helpful as natural sweeteners, particularly raisins and dates, but do try to obtain fruit that has not been treated with chemicals. The sulphur dioxide used to preserve dried fruits destroys vitamin B_1 (thiamine) in the body and may interact adversely with other chemical additives. Use raisins that are sun-dried and free of all additives, and date chips that come from organic suppliers as snack substitutes for children. If you cannot obtain organically grown sun-dried fruit, be careful to blanch all dried fruit in boiling water and rinse again in cold water before using.

Natural whole brown rice
This is rich in vitamins B and E and contains 300 to 400 percent more of the B vitamins than polished white rice. Try
to obtain organically grown brown rice. It has a far better
flavor and is well worth the extra cost.

Yeast and vegetable extracts
These are excellent to use as spreads or for flavoring soups,
casseroles, or gravies.

Bread
Make every effort to bake your own bread, using the quick
Grant loaf method in the starch recipe section. Although
the sales of "brown" bread have risen in recent years, there
is still much confusion about what is a genuine whole wheat
loaf baked from 100 percent whole wheat flour. If you have
a reliable baker, you can check the ingredients but if you
are not sure, it is far better to be independent! Some of the
chain bakeries produce whole-grain bread, but these loaves
often contain emulsifiers, permitted antioxidants, and fat.
Moreover the whole wheat flour from which the bread is
made is not organically grown. Most good health food shops
are now able to supply whole wheat flour from an organic
source. Good bread, supplying all the naturally occurring
vitamins, minerals, and fiber contained in whole wheat is
absolutely fundamental to good health.

Meat, eggs, and cheese
Happily there is a far greater demand now for meat that
comes from animals raised naturally, without hormones or
antibiotics in their feed. Obviously, beef, lamb, and chicken,
produced by traditional methods, cost more but the meat
tastes much better and, because you need less of it on the
Hay System, the overall cost per week should not be any
greater than the diet of incompatible meals, using more
meat. It is worth making every effort to seek out organic
producers of meat, chickens, eggs, and natural cheeses. *The
Organic Food Guide,* published by the Henry Doubleday Re-

search Association, provides up to date information on where such good foods and fresh fruits and vegetables are to be found. Although fruit and some vegetables will not store, meat *can* be bought in bulk and frozen.

Potatoes

These are a "convenience" food *par excellence.* They help to improve the diet by eliminating the use of too much cereal starch, and they contain more available calcium, phosphorus, iron, and B vitamins than do ground cereals. In the Hay System, they are promoted to a place of honor as a main dish, accompanied by vegetables or salads; suggestions for potato meals are included in the starch recipe section. The most valuable part of the potato lies just below the skin. The average family annually throws away potato peelings equivalent in iron to 500 eggs, in protein to sixty steaks, and in vitamin C to five glasses of orange juice. For this reason, try to obtain a supply of potatoes from an organic grower. They store well in a cool, dark place, so you can buy enough at one time to last through the winter. Better still, if you can, grow your own.

The flavor of organically grown potatoes is far superior to commercially grown ones, and there is no danger that the skins will have been treated with anti-sprouting chemicals. If you are not sure about the origin of the potatoes you buy, make sure that the skins are *very* thoroughly scrubbed before cooking.

Nuts

Buy them in the shell and crack them just before use. In this way, they will store well for some time. Once nuts have been shelled, they should be used as soon as possible because exposure to light turns their fat rancid. They do, however, freeze well.

Nuts are a very concentrated food containing fat and protein. They are unadulterated foods that can replace animal protein. The protein in ¾ ounce of nuts is equal to 1 ounce of meat or fish. Most nuts contain unsaturated fat; the exceptions are coconuts and cashews, whose fat is saturated. All nuts contain carbohydrates as well as fiber. They are best combined with vegetables, salads, or fruits.

One of the most valuable nuts is the almond, which contains practically no starch. It has a fat content of 50 to 55 percent and about 20 percent protein. Almonds are rich in magnesium, iron, and potassium but low in sodium. The almond is classed as an alkaline food.

Other valuable alkaline nuts are hazelnuts and Brazilnuts. The sweet chestnut is also an alkaline food but contains a much greater proportion of starch and little protein or fat. Chestnuts cannot therefore be used to replace meat protein, and should not be combined with protein foods or acid fruits.

Peanuts, which are really a legume (and therefore not recommended), cashews, pecans, and walnuts are acid-forming and all contain valuable amounts of protein. Pecans are particularly valuable because they are very easily digested and therefore are especially good for elderly people. Though expensive, only 1½ ounces are required to replace an average serving of meat. All nuts are a good source of vitamins B and E and contain calcium, phosphorus, and potassium.

Be wary of commercial nut butters, which are usually made from highly roasted nuts and heavily salted. They are usually extremely acid-forming, especially peanut butter.

Seeds
Sunflower, pumpkin, and sesame seeds are excellent sources of protein, and EFA, vitamins, minerals, and trace elements. They are rich in magnesium and calcium. Pumpkin seeds are rich in B vitamins, phosphorus, iron, and zinc. Sesame seeds are particularly rich in calcium and vitamin E. Sunflower seeds are also rich in vitamin E, as well as the B-complex, iron, magnesium, and zinc. In her book, *The Joy of Beauty*, Kenton suggests grinding equal quantities of sunflower, sesame, and pumpkin seeds in a blender and storing them in the refrigerator. Add a spoonful of the mixed

seeds to breakfast dishes. All these seeds make excellent between-meal snacks, too. Buy only what you need for immediate use because they quickly turn rancid when exposed to the air.

Raw foods are vital
Eat as much of your food raw as you possibly can. Aim for at least one salad a day composed of raw fruits, green leaves, and roots and, as far as possible, eat all fruit in its raw state.

Only raw foods yield their full complement of vitamins, minerals, and fiber. Heat immediately reduces and often destroys completely the vitamin C content of fruits and vegetables as well as other valuable elements. Most people have far too little vitamin C in their diet. The body needs a constant daily supply if it is to retain its youthfulness in old age.

Many studies have demonstrated the cleansing and curative effect of raw food on the human organism. In particular, it has been found that cooking destroys valuable enzymes in the plant cells, which help in the digestion of raw food, thus relieving the intestinal tract and ensuring better assimilation. For many years, raw food diets have been used in the Bircher-Benner clinic in Zurich for the treatment of arthritis and other conditions, and fresh raw salads and sprouted seeds and grains are an essential part of the therapeutic diet recommended by the Cancer Help Center in Bristol. The book *Raw Energy*, by Leslie and Susannah Kenton, reviews much of the scientific evidence that demonstrates how problems such as fatigue, stress, hypertension, arthritis, and premature aging can be reduced by adopting a mainly raw food diet and gives much sound, practical advice on how to follow this type of regime.

Sprouted seeds, legumes, and grains
Fresh sprouts are a marvelous way of increasing your intake of vitamins and minerals because germinating seeds and grains increases their nutritional value. The vitamin C content of wheat berries increases 60 percent during sprout-

ing. Sprouts are delicious in salads and are easy to grow in a sprouting tray or jar at any time of the year, so they are especially valuable in winter. The best seeds to sprout are alfalfa, mung beans, aduki beans, lentils, fenugreek, or wheat.

To sprout seeds, take a heaped tablespoon of your chosen seeds or beans and put them into a clean 2-pound jar. Cover them with lukewarm (not hot) water and leave them overnight. Next day, cover the jar with a piece of muslin or cheesecloth and secure it with a rubber band. Then drain off the water and replace it with fresh tepid water, pouring off the excess. The seeds should be rinsed and drained twice a day. The sprouts will be ready to eat when they are between ½ and 2½ inches long, depending on which seed you have used. In *The Raw Food Way to Health* by Janet Hunt there is an excellent chapter on sprouting seeds, including details on how to grow and use a great many different kinds.

Fresh herbs
Try to grow some fresh herbs; if you have no garden, they can be grown in pots on the window sill. Parsley in particular should always be used fresh and it makes a valuable addition to salads, vegetable dishes, and egg dishes. It is particularly high in vitamin C and iron.

The use of herbs in salads and cooking can help to improve flavor, stimulate appetite, and decrease the need for salt in food preparation. Many herbs can be grown easily in a small space:

- Basil is an annual that is delicious in all tomato dishes, tomato salads, with zucchini, and beans. It should be used fresh.

- Winter savory makes a compact bush; the flavor of the leaves enhances all bean dishes.

- Tarragon is delicious in chicken dishes; it's also good in salads and mixes well with other herbs.

- Rosemary, sage, and thyme can all be used dried but they are easy to grow in a small space.

- Chives are a very useful herb for those who don't like a strong onion flavor.

Though not actually herbs, mustard greens and garden cress can be grown easily on the kitchen window sill and they make a valuable addition to salads or sandwiches.

Lamb's lettuce can give another welcome crop of green leaves in winter. Grow it outside, or in pots or boxes on a window sill. Joy Larkcom's helpful and practical book *Salads the Year Round* will help indoor and outdoor gardeners to increase their range of herbs and salad plants.

Blueprint for the Hay System Meal Plan
For most people, the easiest way to follow the Hay System is to make one meal a day consist of alkaline foods only; one meal of protein with a salad, vegetables, and fruit; and one meal of starch foods with a salad, vegetables, and a sweet fruit. The basic meal plan looks something like this:

Breakfast (Alkaline)
Fresh fruit in season—best of all is a well-flavored apple; natural live yogurt, preferably homemade, with a tablespoon of wheat germ; a hot drink such as weak tea, herb tea, maté tea, dandelion coffee, or real coffee (not instant). If coffee is chosen, it should be made from finely ground coffee beans, using the filter method, which keeps back undesirable coffee oils and acids, and served with hot milk (half and half). Coffee should be used in strict moderation. Black coffee is not recommended. Tea and coffee should be made with bottled spring water rather than tap water, and on no account use fluoridated water. In some areas a water filter may be helpful and reduce the cost of bottled water, but they do not filter out fluoride or nitrates from the water supply.

Lunch (Starch)
Potatoes cooked in their skins, butter, cooked vegetables, or a salad; one of the sweet fruits or a dessert from the starch recipe section.

Alternatively this meal may consist of home-baked whole wheat bread with butter and a green salad or just a "salad" sandwich. If bran is taken, it should be included with this meal. It can be mixed with wheat germ, a few raisins, and a little milk. If more convenient, it can be taken with the fruit breakfast, but this is not ideal.

Evening Meal (Protein)
Vegetable soup (made without stock), a moderate portion of meat, fish, chicken, shellfish, eggs, or cheese; a salad of fresh raw vegetables; cooked green and/or root vegetables but not potatoes. This can be followed by fresh fruit from the "acid" class such as apples, pears, oranges, and so on. Do not add sugar to these. Only one protein dish should be served and the helpings should be moderate. When no starches are eaten at this meal, less protein is required and more is digested.

The above meals are interchangeable. If a starch breakfast is preferred, the midday meal can be the alkaline meal. Dr. Hay suggested that very active people should have their protein meal at lunch and the starch meal in the evening because the starchy meal entails more digestion than the protein type. This need not mean cooking at lunch; a simple protein meal could consist of a green salad with natural cheese followed by fresh fruit.

For people who are very sedentary or who have special problems to overcome, it is recommended that the number of alkaline meals should be increased, and the number of meals containing concentrated protein or grain starch should be decreased. The best way to do this is to have *two* alkaline meals a day and have protein or starch for the third meal on alternate days. An alkaline meal based on potatoes can be very valuable in these circumtances to replace the grain starch meal.

Points to Remember
Finally, the following points are important to remember when starting to put the Hay System into practice:

- Avoid eating between meals. If you feel you *must* eat something, try sunflower seeds. As well as being very good to eat, they are an extremely rich source of protein, minerals, amino acids, enzymes, and vitamins A, B-complex, D, E, and F.

- If doing without sugar is difficult at first, use a teaspoon or so of "honey syrup" made by dissolving one tablespoon of honey in a half cup of boiled and cooled water. Store this in a screw-top jar. On no account should artificial sweeteners be used; they can quickly destroy vitamin C and eventually may cause liver damage.

- Don't drink unless thirsty, and not immediately before or after meals. If desired, a cup of weak herb or maté tea, with lemon or a small teaspoon of honey, can be taken in the afternoon. Once you are established on a correct meal pattern, snacks of sweets will no longer be appealing.

- Eat fresh vegetables, salads, and fruits as freely as possible.

- Never eat when you are tired or mentally upset.

- Treat alcohol with great respect; it should be used in strict moderation. Don't drink sweet wines, sweet sherry, liqueurs, and sugary cocktails. A good dry wine, however, is compatible with a protein meal and helps digestion. Whisky and gin are "neutral" but beer is classed as a "refined carbohydrate" and should be avoided at (or near) a protein meal.

- Above all, don't forget that however important it is to eat the right foods, exercise and rest, fresh air and sunshine, deep breathing and *positive thinking* are all essential to health.

7.
MENU PLANNING AND SUGGESTIONS

The menus and recipes that follow are from the authors' personal collections and are not intended to be comprehensive. No recipes for roasts or grilled meat are included as these can be found in any standard cookbook. Nor will you find any recipes for cakes, cookies, or fried foods—the items that contribute so much fat, much of it "hidden," to our modern diet. You *will* find that our recipes use butter and cream but the amounts are small, and because the use of meat and milk is restricted, the consumption of saturated fats is automatically reduced.

The recipes themselves contain only compatible ingredients and all the recipes in each section are compatible with each other, so that a correctly combined main meal can be assembled from the protein *or* the starch section. However, it is very important to plan your meals for the day so that alkaline foods always predominate.

In his book *Building Better Bodies*, Dr. Hay listed foods in the following order of importance:

1. Fruits
2. Leafy greens and raw salad foods
3. Root vegetables
4. Grains
5. Proteins

He maintained that we need protein in only very small quantities and that all the elements for human health can be supplied by fruits, greens, roots, and milk. He contended that meat, eggs, and even cereal foods are not essential and in large quantities they can over-stimulate and overburden the metabolism. He also stressed that complex dishes should be avoided and that the best meals are composed of simple dishes of unprocessed foods and limited to two or three items. So, although it is possible to compile a three- or four-course dinner menu from the protein section, it is better to plan the main meal of the day around a *single* main dish of *either* protein *or* starch with a salad and fresh vegetables, followed by just a piece of fresh acid or sweet fruit. The dessert recipes are intended only for occasional use.

The seasonal menu plans have been compiled to show how the Hay System works over a week or so of family meal planning, and include suggestions for breakfasts, main meals without meat, very simple or fast meals that are easy to prepare when time is short or you are feeling tired, meals that use leftovers, and meals for entertaining. If you are the only Hay dieter in the family, you can still follow the system but supplement the meals of non-Hay people with items that you yourself do not have, such as potatoes with meat meals. When entertaining or eating out, it is best to plan your menu around a protein main dish. People won't even notice, if there are several different vegetables, that you haven't helped yourself to bread or potatoes, and at home you can plan a compatible dessert. If cornered, as it were, when eating out, simply ignore the dessert or any other item that is not compatible with your main course. In the words of Surgeon Captain Cleave, author of *The Saccharine Disease*, "If you don't want it, don't eat it."

About kitchen equipment: make sure that your cooking pans are *not* made of aluminum, which can produce chronic aluminum poisoning. If possible use stainless steel—though expensive it lasts a lifetime—Pyrex, or Corningware. Similarly, if using aluminum foil for roasting, use it only as an *outer* wrapping, after the food has been wrapped in buttered waxed paper, because of the danger of aluminum contamination.

Freezing
Because many of the recipes are low in fat or use raw or only lightly cooked vegetables, most of them are not suitable for freezing. If a dish will freeze well, we have mentioned it in the recipe.

Seasonal Menus
The following menus make use of each season's fruits and vegetables as much as possible because this still makes sense in terms of what our bodies need at different times of the year. The meal plan allows for one main meal per day and one light meal in addition to breakfast. Lunches and dinners are interchangeable and the menu for lunch on Sunday allows for entertaining.

A = Alkaline
P = Protein
S = Starch

SPRING MENUS FOR ONE WEEK

	Breakfast	Lunch	Dinner
Sunday	A Grapefruit sections	P Roast Chicken with Wheat Germ Stuffing (page 167) Savory Mushrooms (page 175) Celery Root Purée (page 173) Fruit and Raspberry Dessert (page 178)	S Mixed Vegetable Soup (page 195) Oatcakes (page 227) and butter
Monday	A Orange sections and yogurt	P Sack lunch: Cold chicken slices between lettuce leaves Leftover Mixed Vegetable Soup in thermos Fruit of choice	S Potatoes Dauphinois á la Hay (page 213) Green salad Dried date chips or soaked, dried figs
Tuesday	A Spiced Apple and Raisin Pudding (page 180) and yogurt	S Salad sandwiches Banana and sunflower seeds	P Celery, Apple, and Raisin Salad with slices of natural cheddar cheese

Wednesday	**A** Soaked dried apricots and yogurt	**P** Cottage cheese with tossed green salad Pineapple Yogurt (page 186)	**S** Rice Pilaff (page 209) White mustard greens and garden cress Banana Cream (page 220)
Thursday	**A** Spiced Apple and Raisin Pudding (page 180) and yogurt	**S** Mushrooms on toast White mustard greens and garden cress Dates	**P** Grilled flounder Parsley butter Steamed broccoli spears
Friday	**A** Sliced banana with wheat germ and yogurt	**S** Pecan and Pasta Salad (page 200) Oatcakes (page 227) and butter	**P** Leek Salad (page 143) Vegetables with Ground Beef (page 160) Apricot Mousse (page 182)
Saturday	**A** Bircher Muesli (page 119)	**P** Stuffed Eggs (page 163) Coleslaw (page 142) Fresh fruit of choice	**S** Baked Potatoes with Mushroom Filling (page 215) Green salad Frozen Bananas (page 223)

SUMMER MENUS FOR ONE WEEK

	Breakfast	Lunch	Dinner
Sunday	A Fresh raspberries Yogurt	P Tomato and Parsley Cup (page 135) Chicken with Lemon (page 158) Zucchini Deluxe (page 171) Green salad Sliced Nectarines in a Glass (page 182)	S Creamed Mushrooms on whole wheat toast Date Ice Cream (page 221)
Monday	A Black currants with honey and yogurt	S Eggplant Pâté (page 203) on toast (or in sandwiches) Nuts and raisins	P Zucchini and Tarragon Soup (page 134) Cold chicken Lettuce and green salad Sliced fresh apricots
Tuesday	A Sliced fresh apricots with yogurt	P Green salad with sliced cheddar cheese	S Whole wheat Pasta Shells with Parsley Sauce (page 207) Frozen Bananas (page 223)

Wednesday	**A** Fresh sliced peach with yogurt	**P** Tabouli (page 199) Watercress Fresh grapes	**S** Creamed Cauliflower Cheese (page 165) Tomato Salad with Fresh Basil (page 144) Cherries
Thursday	**A** Raspberries and red currants with yogurt	**P** Mixed vegetable salad with Farmer's cheese Cherries	**S** New potatoes baked with butter and parsley Garden peas and sliced zucchini Baked honey custard
Friday	**A** Sliced fresh apricots with yogurt	**S** Sack lunch: Sandwiches of salad greens and Savory Butter (page 229) Dates	**P** Grilled lemon sole and parsley butter Grilled tomatoes Green salad Raspberry and red currant compote with cream
Saturday	**A** Fresh strawberries with yogurt	**S** Fava bean and Savory Salad (page 200) Whole wheat rolls with cream cheese	**P** Spanish Omelet (page 162) Green salad Fresh peaches

AUTUMN MENUS FOR ONE WEEK

		Breakfast	Lunch	Dinner
Sunday		A Sliced apples and raisins with yogurt	P Roast topside of beef Cauliflower and brussels sprouts Carrot and White Beet Salad (page 147) Baked Stuffed Apples with Cream (page 181)	S Baked Potatoes with Crispy Skins (page 217) Green salad Dates and nuts
Monday		S Uncooked rolled oats with sliced bananas and milk	A Coleslaw (page 142) Pears and yogurt	P Cold roast beef Top Favorite All-seasons Salad (page 138) Sliced oranges
Tuesday		A Sliced apple and yogurt sprinkled with wheat germ	P Waldorf Salad (page 142) Stewed apricots	S Potato Cakes (page 217) Ratatouille (page 170) (enough for two meals) Fresh figs

Day	A		
Wednesday	Sliced pear and yogurt	**S** Sack lunch: Salad sandwiches with Savory Butter (page 229) Bananas	**P** Broiled lamb chops Ratatouille (page 170) Green salad Russet apples and walnuts
Thursday	Sliced apple and yogurt sprinkled with wheat germ	**P** Cream of celery soup Cottage cheese and orange salad	**S** Vegetable Casserole (page 211) Dates and nuts
Friday	Sliced grapefruit and yogurt sprinkled with grated hazelnuts	**S** Sack lunch: Garden Cress and cream cheese sandwiches Very sweet grapes	**P** Grilled mackerel Green salad Frozen Strawberry Mousse (page 179)
Saturday	Sliced pear and yogurt	**P** Avocado Salad á la Guacamole (page 141) with cheddar cheese Apple and Raisin Pudding (page 181) with cream	**S** Spaghetti with Pesto (page 206) Ginger Bananas (page 221)

WINTER MENUS FOR ONE WEEK

	Breakfast	Lunch	Dinner
Sunday	A Fresh grapefruit and orange sections	P Endive, Walnut, and Lamb's Lettuce Salad (page 146) Roast lamb Brussels sprouts Celery Root Purée (page 173) Fresh pineapple slices	S Potato Soup (page 194) Oatcakes (page 227) with butter
Monday	A Shredded raw apple with wheat germ and yogurt	S Baked potatoes with butter White mustard greens and garden cress Sliced tomato	P Leek and Cauliflower Soup (page 131) Cold roast lamb Red Cabbage, Apple, and Hazelnut Salad (page 145) Sliced oranges
Tuesday	S Cooked Oatmeal (page 228) with milk	A Mixed Vegetable Soup (page 195) Carrot and Raisin Salad (page 201)	P Creamed Cauliflower Cheese (page 165) Green salad with sprouted seeds Fresh fruit

	A	P / S	S / P
Wednesday	Soaked dried apricots with wheat germ and yogurt	**P** Sack lunch: Celery Root Soup (page 193), Cheddar Cheese, Apples	**S** Rice with Leeks and Cashew Nuts (page 208), White mustard greens and garden cress, Sliced banana with sesame seeds
Thursday	Sliced apple and raisins with yogurt	**P** Mixed green salad, Individual herb omelet, Oranges	**S** Vegetable Casserole (page 211), Buttered Cabbage (page 174), Fresh grapes
Friday	Soaked dried figs with wheat germ and yogurt	**S** Banana and Date Salad (page 202), Whole wheat bread and butter	**P** Oven Baked Sole (page 155), Savory Mushrooms (page 175), Green salad, Apricot and Apple Fool (page 181)
Saturday	Bircher Muesli (page 119)	**P** Celery, Apple, and Raisin Salad (page 143) with Almond Balls (page 166)	**S** Hazelnut Roast (page 212), Bean sprout and lettuce salad

Main Meals Without Meat
The alkaline and starch meals present no problems for the vegetarian but the following suggestions for protein main meals without meat may be helpful.

- Spanish Omelet (page 161)
  Green salad with French dressing
  Fresh fruit

- Avocado Salad á la Guacamole (page 140), served with thin slices of cheddar cheese
  Fresh pears (peeled and sliced), served with Apricot Sauce (page 189) and sprinkled with toasted sesame seeds

- Stuffed Eggs (page 163)
  Leek Salad (page 142)
  Baked Stuffed Apples (page 182) with cream

- Thick Mixed Vegetable Soup (page 195), topped with grated cheese
  Fresh fruit

- Almond Balls (page 166)
  Coleslaw (page 141)
  Pineapple Yogurt (page 187) or fresh fruit

- Creamed Cauliflower Cheese (page 165)
  Top Favorite All-seasons Salad (page 138)
  Frozen Strawberry Mousse (page 180)

- Waldorf Salad (page 141)
  Hot Apple and Raisin Pudding (page 182) with cream

Breakfasts
Breakfast should always be a light meal. Dr. Hay regarded it as superfluous, but if this seems too drastic, limit breakfast to a light meal of fresh fruit only or fresh fruit and milk or yogurt. This provides the alkaline meal that is so important. If however you prefer a starch breakfast, this can be based on fresh whole cereals and sweet fruits.

Suggestions for both types of meal are listed below:

Alkaline Breakfasts
- Any fresh acid fruit in season (see compatible food chart) with milk or yogurt
- Fresh grapefruit or orange juice
- Grated apple with one tablespoon of wheat germ and yogurt
- Sliced fresh fruit and yogurt, topped with sunflower seeds
- Soaked dried apricots with yogurt and one tablespoon of wheat germ

Note: Bran and wheat germ may be added to the alkaline breakfast if desired. They are regarded as neutral because their starch content is negligible.

Muesli
Muesli is now a very popular breakfast dish, but unfortunately the commercial "muesli" mix bears no relationship at all to the original raw fruit porridge devised by Dr. Max Bircher-Benner for his patients. Modern mueslis are essentially starchy cereal mixes whereas in Dr. Bircher-Benner's muesli, grated raw apple or other acid fruit predominated and only a *level tablespoon* of fresh rolled oats or medium oatmeal was permitted. Because the cereal content is so small and also because it is raw, freshly made muesli, prepared according to Dr. Bircher-Benner's recipe, may be regarded as an alkaline meal. The recipe is given below. However, if you prefer a *mixed cereal* dish, this is *not* muesli and should be regarded as a starch meal to be combined with one of the sweet fruits.

Dr. Bircher-Benner's Muesli
1 *level* tablespoon rolled oats or medium oatmeal
3 tablespoons water

1 tablespoon lemon juice
3 tablespoons raw milk if obtainable or natural yogurt
2 medium apples
1 tablespoon grated almonds or hazelnuts

1. Soak the oats or oatmeal in the water overnight.

2. In the morning, add the lemon juice, grate the well-scrubbed apples into the mixture, and sprinkle the grated nuts on top.

3. Serve at once.

Starch Breakfasts
- A helping of mixed raw cereals (such as a muesli base), topped with one tablespoon of wheat bran and two teaspoons of raisins, soaked in three tablespoons of water overnight, and served with milk

- Whole wheat toast with butter and a little honey

- Poached or scrambled egg yolks on whole wheat toast

- Millet flakes with sliced bananas and milk

- Homemade cooked oatmeal

- Soaked dried figs with mixed whole cereals and milk

- Uncooked rolled oats, soaked overnight, and served with sliced banana and milk

Note: All cereal dishes may have bran and/or wheat germ added to them if desired.

Practical Suggestions for Special Problems
Special health problems have been discussed in Part One, but those who are tackling the following conditions may find these suggestions helpful:

Allergies

When adopting the Hay System, allergy sufferers may find it easier *at first* to continue omitting the foods to which they are intolerant. If they are attending an allergy clinic, a recently published booklet, *What Can I Eat?*, will be helpful. The author, Pearl Coleman, is a well-known writer on health topics.

As allergy sufferers become established on a diet of compatible foods, however, they will find very quickly that they are no longer intolerant of any good, unprocessed food, or of natural substances in the environment.

Arthritis

The diet of arthritis sufferers should have a comprehensive vitamin and mineral supplement. There are, however, three outstanding needs:

Vitamin C: This stimulates the production of hydrocortisone, the chief hormone where arthritis is concerned, and is also related to the nutrition of the joints.

Pantothenic acid (B5): Like vitamin C, this is vital to the normal production of cortisone and other adrenal hormones. According to Dr. Roger Williams – the first scientist to identify, isolate, and synthesize pantothenic acid – it may be important in *preventing* arthritis.

Cod liver oil: This not only supplies vitamins A and D and iodine, but also furnishes the means necessary for fixing calcium in the body. Take a tablespoon daily, on an empty stomach, an hour before a meal or four hours afterwards. It should also be emulsified for greater effectiveness according to the following instructions:

1. Place one tablespoon of pure, unflavored cod liver oil in a small glass jar (such as a vitamin bottle).
2. Add two tablespoons of freshly squeezed orange juice

(frozen orange juice is not suitable) and shake for a few seconds.

3. Swallow quickly.

Surprisingly, the orange juice completely masks the unpleasant taste of the oil. Milk can be used instead of orange juice but does not mask the taste.

The cod liver oil should be taken daily till the pain subsides, then every second day for the next three months. After that, take once every two weeks, indefinitely. Apart from its beneficial effect on arthritis, it is an excellent tonic for both health and beauty, and retards the aging process.

Indigestion
This condition, as shown in Part One, Chapter Three, subsides rapidly with a diet of compatible meals. But it subsides even more rapidly if a tablespoon of wheat germ is taken at each meal. Wheat germ is an excellent source of the B vitamins, which help digestion and are especially necessary for the digestion of starch foods. Although wheat germ contains the principal part of the protein of grains, the amount of this protein is insignificant. Wheat germ can therefore be taken with any meal.

Sleeplessness
People who suffer from this condition should endeavor to make the last meal of the day as simple as possible, consisting of one course, but an amply satisfying amount. A protein meal is preferable to a starchy one. Coffee and strong tea should be omitted from the diet. Coffee, if insisted upon, should be limited to one cup per day, diluted with milk or cream, and taken in the early part of the day. B vitamins in the form of wheat germ, brewer's yeast, and calcium pantothenate should supplement the diet. Calcium and magnesium are also very helpful.

Overweight

To speed up the process of losing weight, a fruit and milk breakfast should be preferred. A mixture of freshly squeezed orange juice and milk makes a delicious and satisfying drink. This mixture is not indigestible as so many people erroneously believe; the orange juice actually enhances the digestion of the milk.

If you lead an active life the protein meal is best taken at midday, as the starch meal requires more digestion than the protein meal. Only a very moderate helping of the protein dish should be taken but you can also have vegetable soup, salad, and root and/or green vegetables, with fresh fruit to follow.

The starch meal is best based on whole grains or potatoes. Bread in any quantity, and indeed most cereal starches, are best avoided while you are trying to lose weight. A potato meal as described in the starch recipe section, accompanied by a salad and/or green vegetables, is the best kind of starch meal for the overweight.

If you lead a fairly sedentary life, try to have *two* alkaline meals per day, i.e. breakfast as above and lunch or dinner consisting of salad, vegetables, and fruit. Meat should be limited to once or twice a week.

Burping

Food repeats if the combinations of the meal are wrong. If a person has had a habit of burping for a long time, repeating may persist for some time after the combinations have been corrected.

Gas

This indicates that too much acid-forming food has been eaten daily for too long a time. When the body chemistry is even approximately normal, natural foods seldom if ever produce gas. This condition will quickly disappear when foods are correctly combined.

The Alkaline Meal
Because the alkaline foods should predominate in the diet, they are an essential part of *every* meal in the form of the salads, vegetables, and fruits that accompany protein or starch dishes. However, the easiest time to fit in a wholly alkaline meal is usually at breakfast and suggestions for this meal are in the breakfast section.

Alkaline main meals can be composed of green or root vegetables either steamed or cooked conservatively with a little water and served with a little butter or cream, accompanied by any combination of raw vegetables, sprouted seeds, salad ingredients, and/or fresh acid fruit. Follow with fruit or sunflower seeds. A starch version of the alkaline meal can consist of a baked potato with a little butter, a green salad with a dressing appropriate to a starch meal, and a cooked green vegetable. This can be followed by one of the sweet fruits listed for a starch meal. If, however, a potato meal is taken as the alkaline meal, no other starch meal should be taken that day.

The list of alkali-forming foods at the end of the book will help in assembling wholly alkaline main meals, and the following list of easily prepared salads shows what tremendous variety can be introduced into the concept of the alkaline meal.

Twenty Fruit and Vegetable Salads for Alkaline Meals
• Chopped apple, chives and cabbage

• Grated carrot, apple, and raisins

• Chopped apple and celery with cress

• Grated beets and onion with shredded cabbage

• Grated celery root with sliced red and green peppers

• Sliced tomatoes with chopped fresh basil

• Sliced endive, sliced ripe pears, and watercress

• Shredded white cabbage, apples, and raisins

- Shredded red cabbage and orange sections
- Sprouted alfalfa (or other sprouted seeds), fresh parsley, and chopped leek
- Chopped crisp radishes and sliced cucumber on shredded crisp lettuce
- Fresh peas cooked with mint and served with shredded lettuce and some fresh, chopped tarragon
- Small zucchini grated and served with chopped chives and tarragon on shredded lettuce
- Cauliflower flowerets with cooked peas and sliced green peppers sprinkled with freshly chopped mint
- Diced fresh pineapple with tangerine sections and chopped mint
- Shredded white cabbage, diced pineapple, and sliced green peppers
- Shredded tiny brussels sprouts, diced celery, and sunflower seeds
- Sliced cucumber, lamb's lettuce, and chopped walnuts
- Shredded endive, grapefruit sections, and chopped pecan nuts
- Diced beets, chopped celery, and chopped walnuts

With either Basic French Dressing: three parts oil to one part lemon juice. Shake in a glass jar with sea salt and freshly ground black pepper to taste and a little honey. For extra "bite" add one teaspoon Dijon mustard.

Or sweet cream or sour cream dressing: cream or sour cream seasoned with a little salt and paprika.

Miscellaneous Pointers

Animal fats: Two ounces (50g) per day is believed to be the maximum allowance, and less than this would be advisable. Vegetable fats in the form of salad oil can be added to this allowance.

Melons: These are an excellent food, but are not easily digested with other foods. They are best taken on their own, making an excellent alkaline meal.

Peanut butter: This contains a great deal of starch along with a great deal of protein—as do all the legumes. It is therefore indigestible and acid-forming and is best used very infrequently. There are some delicious nut butters that can be used instead, such as sesame spread, which contains just unhulled sesame seeds and sea salt with no sugar or chemical additives.

Distilled water: Although this may be indicated in certain cases of stones or arthritis, it is not recommended for daily use. It is in what is termed a "nascent state" and, being wholly unsaturated, is ready to take up any chemical with which it comes into contact. The best drinking water is a good spring water that is *not heavily mineralized.*

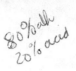 80% alk.
20% acid

TABLE OF COMPATIBLE FOODS

Columns I and III are incompatible

Can be combined   Can be combined

I	II	III
For Protein Meals	**Neutral Foods**	**For Starch Meals**
PROTEINS 1x day	NUTS acid - walnut cashew	GRAINS acid 1x day
Meat of all kinds: Beef, lamb, pork, vension acid	All except peanuts alk - almond	Wholegrain: Wheat, barley, maize (corn), oats, millet,
	FATS chestnut brazilnut	rice (brown, unpolished), rye
Poultry: Chicken, duck, goose, turkey acid	Butter	Bread (100% whole wheat)
	Cream	Flour (100% or 85%)
Game: Pheasant, partridge, grouse, hare acid	Egg yolks	Oatmeal (medium)
	Olive oil (virgin)	
	Sunflower seed oil	
Fish of all kinds including shellfish acid	Sesame seed oil (cold pressed)	
Eggs acid.		
Cheese acid		
Milk (combines best with fruits and should not be served at a meat meal) alk		
Yogurt		
FRUITS alkali	**VEGETABLES** alkali	**SWEET FRUITS** alkali
Apples	All green and root vegetables	Bananas (if ripe)
Apricots (fresh and dried)	except potatoes and	Dates
Blackberries	Jerusalem artichokes	Figs (fresh and dried)
Blueberries	Asparagus	Grapes (extra sweet)
Cherries	Beans (all fresh green beans)	Papaya (if *very* ripe)
Currants (black, red, or white if ripe)	Beets	Pears (if *very* sweet and ripe)
	Broccoli	Currants
Gooseberries (if ripe)	Brussels sprouts	Raisins
Grapefruit	Cabbage	Sultanas
Grapes	Carrots	
Kiwis	Cauliflower	**VEGETABLES** alkali
Lemons	Celery	
Limes	Celery root	Potatoes
Loganberries	Eggplant	Jerusalem artichokes
Mandarin oranges	Kohlrabi	
Mangoes	Leeks	**MILK AND YOGURT**
Melons (best eaten *alone* as a fruit meal)	Mushrooms	
	Onions	Only in moderation
Nectarines	Parsnips	
Oranges	Peas	
Papayas	Rutabagas	
Pears	Spinach	
Pineapples	Squash	
Prunes (for occasional use)	Turnips	
Raspberries	Zucchini	
Strawberries		
Tangerines		

Note: Plums and cranberries
are *not* recommended

Columns I and III are incompatible

Can be combined   Can be combined

I   II   III

For Protein Meals   **Neutral Foods**   **For Starch Meals**

SALAD DRESSINGS   SALAD INGREDIENTS   SALAD DRESSINGS

French dressing made with Avocados   Sweet or sour cream
  oil and lemon juice or Cucumber   Olive oil or cold pressed
  apple cider vinegar   Endive (chicory)   seed oils
Cream dressing   Fennel   Fresh tomato juice with oil
Mayonnaise (homemade)   Garlic   and seasoning
                      Lamb's lettuce
                      Lettuce
                      Peppers, red and green
                      Radishes
                      Scallions
                      Sprouted legumes
                      Sprouted seeds
                      Tomatoes (uncooked)
                      Watercress
                      White mustard greens and
                        garden cress

                      HERBS AND FLAVORINGS

                      Chives
                      Mint
                      Parsley
                      Sage
                      Tarragon
                      Thyme
                      Grated lemon rind
                      Grated orange rind

                      SEEDS

                      Sunflower *neutral*
                      Sesame
                      Pumpkin

                      BRAN

                      Wheat or oat bran
                      Wheat germ

SUGAR SUBSTITUTE   SUGAR SUBSTITUTE   SUGARS *acid*

Diluted frozen orange juice Raisins and raisin juice Brown sugar
                      Honey   Honey (in strict moderation)
FOR VEGETARIANS (but   Maple syrup
  not recommended)

Legumes *acid*
Lentils
Soybeans
Kidney beans
Chick peas (garbanzos)
Butter (lima) beans
Pinto beans

ALCOHOL   ALCOHOL   ALCOHOL

Dry red and white wines   Whisky   Ale
Dry cider   Gin   Beer

PART THREE
RECIPES FOR PROTEIN MEALS

8.

SOUPS AND APPETIZERS

LEEK AND CAULIFLOWER SOUP

Serves 4–6

2 leeks
2 tablespoons butter
1 small cauliflower
⅛ teaspoon ground mace
3 cups water

1. Wash and chop the leeks.
2. Melt the butter in a large pan and add the leeks.
3. Cook gently until the leeks are transparent.
4. Wash the cauliflower and divide into flowerets.
5. Add the cauliflower, mace, and water to the pan and bring to a boil.
6. Reduce the heat and simmer for about 10 minutes until the cauliflower pieces are tender but not soggy.
7. Remove from the heat and blend in a blender until smooth.
8. Return to the pan and reheat. Season to taste.

TOMATO SOUP

Serves 4

1½ pounds tomatoes
3 celery stalks
1 onion
1 medium carrot
2 tablespoons butter
3¾ cups water
1 teaspoon yeast extract
1 bouquet garni (2-3 sprigs parsley, 1
    sprig thyme, 1 bay leaf, and 1
    clove tied in a muslin bag)
Sea salt and freshly ground black
    pepper
A little milk *or* light cream

1. Skin the tomatoes by dipping them into boiling water for a minute, and cut into slices.
2. Wash the celery, onion, and carrot and cut into slices.
3. Melt the butter in a thick-bottomed pan and add the vegetables.
4. Using a wooden spoon, stir the vegetables for about 5 mintues.
5. Add the water, yeast extract, bouquet garni, and tomatoes. Bring to simmering point.
6. Cover the pan and allow to simmer gently for 15–20 minutes.
7. Remove the bouquet garni and strain the liquid or place in a blender and blend until smooth.
8. Return to the pan and reheat.
9. Season to taste and add a little milk or cream.

MUSHROOM SOUP

Serves 4

2 tablespoons butter
1 small onion, chopped
1 medium carrot
1 celery stalk
4 cups large mushrooms
1 heaping teaspoon yeast extract
2½ cups water
Freshly grated nutmeg
Sea salt
Freshly ground black pepper
4 tablespoons heavy cream
1 tablespoon dry sherry (optional)

1. Melt the butter in a large saucepan, add the chopped onion, and cook very gently until golden brown.
2. Wash and slice the carrot, celery, and mushrooms and add to the onion.
3. Add the yeast extract and water and bring to a boil.
4. Turn the heat down to simmering point, cover the pan, and allow to simmer for approximately 15 minutes until the vegetables are just tender.
5. Pour the mixture into a blender and blend for 30 seconds until smooth; return to the pan.
6. Reheat and add a miserly pinch of grated nutmeg (this gives a subtle flavor and also makes the mushroom flavor sing out).
7. Season to taste and just before serving add the cream.
8. For special occasions add a tablespoon of dry sherry.

ZUCCHINI AND TARRAGON SOUP

Serves 4

1 pound zucchini
3 cups water
2–3 sprigs fresh tarragon *or* 1 tea-
    spoon dried tarragon
Sea salt
Freshly ground black pepper
4 tablespoons sour cream

1. Wash and slice the zucchini.
2. Put the water in a large pan and bring to a boil.
3. Put the zucchini and tarragon into the pan, bring back
   to boiling point, and then reduce the heat to a gentle
   simmer.
4. Simmer for about 5 minutes until the zucchini pieces are
   just tender, but the outside skin retains its bright green
   color.
5. Remove from the heat and blend in a blender for 30 seconds until *almost* smooth but the green flecks of skin
   are still visible.
6. Return to the pan and reheat. Season to taste.
7. Pour into soup bowls and stir a tablespoon of sour cream
   into each bowl. This soup is equally delicious hot or cold.

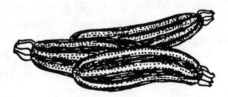

MINTED GRAPEFRUIT

Serves 4

2 large grapefruits
A small handful fresh mint leaves
2 level teaspoons honey

1. Cut the grapefruits into halves and loosen each segment with a grapefruit knife. Remove all pith from the center of each half.
2. Wash, dry, and finely chop the mint leaves.
3. Mix the mint with the honey and place a half teaspoon in the center of each half grapefruit.
4. Place the grapefruit halves in individual serving dishes and chill for 30 minutes.

TOMATO AND PARSLEY CUP

Serves 4

4 large *or* 8 small tomatoes
Fresh parsley
Sea salt
Freshly ground black pepper
A little fresh basil

1. Skin and slice the tomatoes.
2. Wash, dry, and chop the parsley.
3. Mix the tomatoes and parsley (use a generous amount) and season with salt, pepper, and a teaspoon of freshly chopped basil. Use a pinch of dried basil if you have no fresh available.
4. Serve in individual cups.

MUSHROOMS IN SOUR CREAM

Serves 4

1 large tomato
⅔ cup sour cream
1 teaspoon lemon juice
1 tablespoon finely chopped parsley
4 cups small button mushrooms
Sea salt
Freshly ground black pepper
Paprika

1. Peel the tomato and chop finely, removing the seeds.
2. Stir the tomato, lemon juice, and chopped parsley into the sour cream.
3. Wash and dry the mushrooms and slice them.
4. Stir the mushrooms into the cream mixture and season to taste.
5. Spoon the mixture into individual bowls and dust with a very light sprinkling of paprika.
6. Chill for 30 minutes before serving.

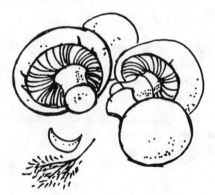

ZUCCHINI VINAIGRETTE

Serves 4

8 small zucchini
1 teaspoon sea salt
1 large onion
6 tablespoons olive oil
3 tablespoons cider vinegar
½ teaspoon Dijon mustard
½ teaspoon clear honey
Paprika
1 tablespoon chopped parsley

1. Wash the zucchini and slice into rounds about ¼ inch thick.
2. Put a little water and sea salt into a saucepan and bring to a boil.
3. Add the zucchini and allow to simmer gently for about 5 minutes until just tender but not soggy.
4. Drain well and allow to cool.
5. Slice the onion finely and arrange with zucchini in individual bowls.
6. Mix the oil, vinegar, Dijon mustard, and honey and pour over the zucchini.
7. Sprinkle each bowl with a pinch of paprika and the chopped parsley.
8. Chill for 30 minute before serving.

9.
SALADS, DRESSINGS, AND SAUCES

TOP FAVORITE ALL-SEASONS SALAD

Serves 4

4 tablespoons Basic French Dressing
(page 148)
4 cups shredded white cabbage
Other ingredients in quantities according to taste:
1 red or green pepper
1–2 celery stalks
Freshly shelled walnuts *or* cashews *or*
freshly skinned almonds
3–4 extra-sweet, dried apricots
1–2 apples
1 small piece of cooked beet
Chives *or* grated onion

1. Place the Basic French Dressing in a large salad bowl.
2. Cut the cabbage into thin shreds and mix with the French Dressing. (Cabbage is the best source of dietary fiber next to wheat bran.) This should be the base of the salad.
3. Skin and slice the pepper, chop the celery, and add to the salad.
4. Add the nuts and dried apricots, both blanched and cut into thin strips.

5. Lastly cut up the apples, leaving the skin on if it is free from chemical sprays, dice the beet, and either chop the chives finely or grate the onion.
6. Mix all the ingredients together well, adding more dressing if necessary. The small piece of beet will give the salad a beautiful pink color.

Variations: The ingredients of this salad can be varied according to season but the base of the salad should always be the cabbage. The apple, too, is a vital ingredient. Infinite variety can be achieved by adding one or more of the following:

• Shredded Florence fennel root

• Young garden peas

• Sprouted seeds or mung beans

• Chopped cucumber

• Chopped mint leaves

• Sliced radishes

• Dried or fresh herbs

• Raisins

• Roughly chopped watercress

• Fresh tarragon (superb!), snipped into small pieces

• Parsley, snipped into small pieces

• Carrot, cut into matchsticks or coarsely grated for speed

• Chopped celery root

• Quartered orange sections

• White mustard greens and garden cress

The secret of a successful salad of this kind is to have as much variety in the texture of the ingredients and in the sizes of shredding as possible. It is important to be able to see the various ingredients and not to reduce the salad to an indistinguishable mush. Some shredding can be done with a sharp knife; other shredding is more effective done with a stainless steel grater that has three different grades of shredding; some ingredients, such as chives and parsley, are best just snipped with kitchen cooking scissors.

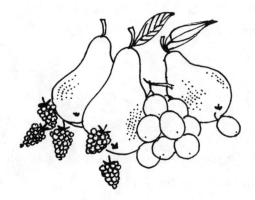

AVOCADO SALAD À LA GUACAMOLE

Serves 4

2 large avocados
Juice of 1 lemon
2 tomatoes
2 celery stalks
½ red pepper, skinned
½ onion *or* 1 shallot
1 clove garlic
2 teaspoons finely chopped parsely
2 tablespoons heavy cream
Sea salt
Freshly ground black pepper

1. Halve the avocadoes lengthwise. Remove the pits and scoop out the inner flesh leaving some adhering to the skin so that there is a thick firm shell remaining.
2. Rub a little of the lemon juice on the inner surface of the shells to prevent discoloration.
3. Cut the scooped-out flesh into cubes, place in a bowl, and stir in the rest of the lemon juice.
4. Skin, deseed, and chop the tomatoes.
5. Chop the celery, red pepper, and onion and add these ingredients and the tomatoes to the avocado in the bowl.
6. Add the garlic, squeezed through a press, parsley, cream, and seasoning.
7. Combine the mixture well; it will thicken and make its own salad dressing.
8. Fill the shells and chill before serving.

Note: This salad makes a refreshing appetizer for 6 people if smaller helpings are served in individual bowls.

Variation
Alternatively, this salad can be served with thin slices of

cheddar cheese as a main course for 4, as a light lunch or evening meal.

WALDORF SALAD

Serves 4–6

4 celery stalks
½ cup chopped walnuts
2 large eating apples
1½ cups cheddar cheese
⅔ cup Mayonnaise (page 151)
Sea salt and freshly ground black
pepper to taste

1. Chop the celery and walnuts.
2. Dice the apples and cheese.
3. Mix all together in a salad bowl and add the Mayonnaise.
4. Give a final mix, adding salt and pepper to taste.

COLESLAW

Serves 4–6

12 ounces white cabbage
8 ounces carrots
1 small onion
⅓ cup seedless raisins
1⅓ cups Mayonnaise (page 151)

1. Shred the cabbage, grate the carrots, and chop the onion finely.
2. Combine all the ingredients in a salad bowl, add the Mayonnaise and toss well. For a lighter coleslaw, toss with Basic French Dressing (page 148).

LEEK SALAD

Serves 4

2 large leeks
1 small green pepper
1 cup walnuts
Sea salt
Freshly ground black pepper
6 tablespoons Basic French Dressing
   (page 148)

1. Trim and clean the leeks thoroughly and slice across finely.
2. Blanch the leeks in boiling water for 2 minutes, drain thoroughly, and allow to cool.
3. Remove the core and seeds from the green pepper and slice finely.
4. Chop the walnuts.
5. Combine the leeks, green pepper, and walnuts in a salad bowl and toss with the dressing.

CELERY, APPLE, AND RAISIN SALAD

Serves 4

1 head celery
2 red-skinned eating apples
⅓ cup raisins
6 tablespoons Basic Sour Cream
   Dressing (page 150)

1. Wash the celery thoroughly and slice finely.
2. Scrub the apples *very* thoroughly and slice.
3. Combine all the ingredients together and toss well with the dressing.

TOMATO SALAD WITH FRESH BASIL

Serves 4

The success of this salad depends on using the finest ingredients: if possible the large beefsteak tomatoes, *fresh* basil, and the best quality olive oil.

> 1 pound large well-flavored tomatoes
> 1 clove garlic
> 2–3 scallions
> A good handful fresh basil leaves
> 6 tablespoons Basic French Dressing
> made with cider vinegar and virgin
> olive oil (page 148)

1. Peel and slice the tomatoes and arrange in a serving dish that has been rubbed with the cut clove of garlic.
2. Chop the scallions very finely and scatter over the tomatoes.
3. Chop the basil leaves finely and sprinkle over the tomatoes and onions.
4. Pour on the French Dressing and leave for 10 minutes for the flavors to blend.

Note: Do not make this salad too far in advance or the tomatoes will become mushy.

RED CABBAGE, APPLE, AND HAZELNUT SALAD

Serves 4

1 pound red cabbage
2 eating apples
⅓ cup raisins
4 tablespoons Basic French Dressing
  (page 148)
⅓ cup coarsely chopped hazelnuts

1. Wash the cabbage and shred finely.
2. Core and chop the apples coarsely.
3. Combine the cabbage, apples, and raisins in a salad bowl, pour on the dressing, and mix well.
4. Sprinkle chopped hazelnuts on the salad just before serving.

Note: This salad is best made between 1 and 2 hours before it is needed.

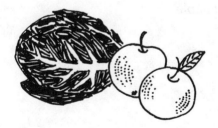

ENDIVE, WALNUT, AND LAMB'S LETTUCE SALAD

Serves 4

1 pound endive
3 heads lamb's lettuce
½ cup coarsely chopped, fresh walnuts
4 tablespoons Basic French Dressing
   made with virgin olive oil (page
   148)

1. Wash the endive and the lamb's lettuce and dry carefully.
2. Slice the endive and place in a bowl with the walnuts.
3. Pour on the French Dressing and turn the pieces in the
   dressing so that they are well coated.
4. Arrange the lamb's lettuce leaves on a serving dish and
   pile the endive and walnuts in the center. Pour on the
   remaining dressing and serve immediately.

Note: This is a salad for gardeners, as I have never seen
lamb's lettuce in a produce department. However, it is a
marvelous winter standby, providing flowerets of small
green leaves throughout the coldest winter. I always plant
it in August to be sure of some salad greens when nothing
else is available.

CARROT AND WHITE BEET SALAD

Serves 4

1¾ cups grated raw white beet
1¾ cups grated carrot
3 tablespoons finely chopped parsley
⅔ cup Basic Sour Cream Dressing
   (page 150)
Sea salt
Freshly ground black pepper

1. Mix the grated white beet and carrot together and add the parsley.
2. Pour on the Basic Sour Cream Dressing and check for seasoning. Add extra salt and pepper if needed.

Note: This is another salad for keen gardeners! Having hated dark red beets since childhood, mainly because their juice usually clashed with the color of tomatoes, I experimented with the white and golden beet varieties (seeds are available through mail-order catalogs from growers specializing in unusual varieties) with great success.

Variation
The golden variety of beet is particularly attractive and this salad could also be made with equal quantities of grated golden beet and apple with a few raisins, using the Basic Sour Cream Dressing.

BASIC FRENCH DRESSING

1 level teaspoon sea salt
½–1 crushed clove of garlic (optional)
1 teaspoon Dijon mustard
2 tablespoons freshly squeezed
  lemon juice *or* cider vinegar
Freshly ground black pepper
6 tablespoons virgin olive oil *or* cold
  pressed sunflower seed oil

1. Put all the ingredients into a screw-top jar and shake vigorously.
2. This amount should be enough to dress two salads or more and can be stored in the refrigerator.
3. If a sweeter dressing is preferred, 1 teaspoon of clear honey can be added to the basic dressing. If garlic is not liked, chopped chives can add an extra zest.

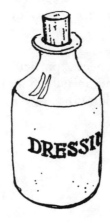

FAVORITE "SWEET-SOUR" DRESSING

    1 small shallot *or* onion
    1 small clove garlic, halved
    1 teaspoon cider vinegar
    1 teaspoon lemon juice
    1 rounded teaspoon honey
    1 teaspoon dry mustard
    *½ cup fresh red pepper, cut up
    ½ cup sunflower seed oil *or* olive oil
    1 pinch dried thyme *or* the equiva-
      lent fresh thyme
    2–3 sprigs of parsley
    1 pinch sea salt

1. In a blender, or a food processor fitted with the steel blade, place all the ingredients except the oil, and start the blending.
2. Then add the oil slowly through the feeder and blend till the mixture is smooth and of the consistency of thin mayonnaise.
3. Adjust the seasoning if necessary and store in the refrigerator in a screw-top glass jar till required.
4. It saves work to make double this quantity, as it keeps well when refrigerated.

*This is an important ingredient.

BASIC SOUR CREAM DRESSING

⅔ cup sour cream
1 teaspoon finely chopped onion *or*
   chives
2 tablespoons lemon juice
1 teaspoon dry mustard
1 teaspoon honey

1. Place all the ingredients in a blender and blend well.

Variations
Yogurt can be used instead of sour cream but is not as effective.

For dressing cabbage salads, the addition of a half teaspoon of yeast extract gives an extra zest.

MAYONNAISE

2 egg yolks at room temperature
1 teaspoon dry mustard
1 pinch sea salt
Freshly ground black pepper
2 tablespoons cider vinegar
1⅓ cups cold pressed olive oil
1 tablespoon boiling water

1. Put the egg yolks and seasoning into a blender.
2. Add the cider vinegar and blend at the lowest speed.
3. Pour the oil into the egg mixture *very slowly* (almost drop by drop) keeping the blender at its lowest speed.
4. Continue to add oil very slowly until the mixture begins to thicken.
5. When the mixture has thickened, add the rest of the oil in a steady stream until it is all incorporated.
6. Lastly, add the boiling water and switch the blender off.

EGGLESS MAYONNAISE*

1 cup whipping cream
1 teaspoon clear honey
¼ teaspoon paprika
½ teaspoon sea salt
1 cup sunflower oil
2 teaspoons lemon juice

1. Whip the cream until soft and fold in the honey, paprika, and salt.
2. Using an electric mixer at slow speed, gradually add the sunflower seed oil.
3. When the mixture begins to thicken, add the lemon juice.

*With acknowledgment to *Tempting and Nutritious Recipes* (Natural Food Associates, Atlanta)

PAPRIKA DRESSING

1 tablespoon fresh lemon juice
3 tablespoons virgin olive oil *or* cold
  pressed sunflower seed oil
1 teaspoon clear, mild honey
1 good pinch paprika
1 tiny pinch cayenne (optional)
1 level teaspoon any herb mixture
  preferred
Sea salt
Freshly ground black pepper

1. Place all the ingredients in a screw-top jar and screw lid on firmly.
2. Shake vigorously before using.

FRESH TOMATO SAUCE

1 medium onion
1 pound fresh tomatoes, beefsteak if
  possible
2 tablespoons butter
1½ cups vegetable stock
1 crushed garlic clove
1 tablespoon tomato paste
1 small handful chopped, fresh basil
  leaves
Sea salt
Freshly ground black pepper

1. Chop the onion; skin and chop the tomatoes.
2. Melt the butter in a large, thick-bottomed pan and cook
   the onion gently until transparent.
3. Add the remaining ingredients and bring to a boil.
4. Reduce the heat and simmer for 20 minutes or so. Do
   not cover the pan.
5. Adjust the seasoning if necesssary.

Note: This is a good standby and can be stored in the refrigerator, or if you have a glut of home-grown tomatoes, it can
be made up in larger quantities as it freezes well.

RED PEPPER SAUCE

2 cups red pepper, deseeded and
   roughly chopped
2–3 large, unpeeled garlic cloves
6 tablespoons virgin olive oil *or* cold
   pressed sunflower seed oil
2 teaspoons lemon juice
Sea salt
Freshly ground black pepper

1. Place the red peppers and garlic in a saucepan with just
   sufficient water to cover and simmer for about 10 minutes
   until the peppers are very tender.
2. Drain, skin the garlic cloves, and blend the peppers and
   garlic in a blender or food processor for a minute or so.
3. With the motor still running at low speed, add the oil
   in drops, slowly, until the mixture has thickened, followed by the lemon juice.

Note: An excellent sauce for serving over skinned and sliced
avocados. Slice these longways to make an attractive presen-
tation. Can be used as a colorful appetizer for special occasions.

10.

MAIN DISHES

OVEN BAKED SOLE

Serves 2

Allow one medium sole for each person. Ask the fish dealer to skin the fish.

> 2 medium soles, skinned but left on
> the bone
> 2 tablespoons butter
> ¼ cup dry white wine
> ¼ cup water *or* fish stock
> Juice of ½ lemon

1. Preheat the oven to 350°.
2. Season the fish and place in a well-buttered ovenproof dish.
3. Pour the wine, water/stock, and lemon juice over the fish.
4. Bake for 15 minutes, basting from time to time.
5. Brown under a very hot broiler for 2 minutes.

156 Food Combining for Health

MACKEREL WITH SORREL OR GOOSEBERRY SAUCE

Buy small, absolutely fresh fish; clean them and score each side of the backbone three times with a sharp knife to allow the heat to reach the thickest part. Cook under a hot broiler, allowing 4–7 minutes for each side. Place on a serving dish and keep warm while finishing the sauce.

Sorrel Sauce
Serves 4

> 1 large handful sorrel leaves
> 2 tablespoons butter
> ⅔ cup light cream
> ⅔ cup heavy cream
> Juice from cooking fish
> Sea salt and freshly ground black
>   pepper

1. Remove the stems from the sorrel and wash thoroughly.
2. Place the leaves and butter in a heavy saucepan and let the leaves simmer gently in the melted butter until they are reduced to a purée (3–4 minutes).
3. In another saucepan, heat the cream but do not let it boil. Stir in the sorrel purée and fish stock, made by adding a little water to the pan in which the mackerel were broiled, and bringing to a boil.
4. Season to taste and serve with the mackerel.

Gooseberry Sauce
Serves 4

This is the classic sauce for mackerel.

1. Follow the above method substituting a purée of ripe sweet gooseberries for the sorrel. Use 2 cups of gooseberries, washed and simmered with a little butter until they are soft enough to purée in a blender.

POACHED FRESHWATER TROUT WITH CREAM AND PARSLEY SAUCE

Serves 4

4 trout
10 cups water
6 tablespoons wine vinegar
2 bay leaves
10 black peppercorns

For the cream and parsley sauce:

4 tablespoons unsalted butter
⅔ cup heavy cream
Sea salt
Freshly ground black pepper
1 tablespoon finely chopped parsley

1. Clean the trout as quickly as possible but don't rinse them.
2. In a large pan, bring water and wine vinegar to a boil and add the bay leaves and peppercorns.
3. To serve hot, slip the trout into the boiling water and simmer 5–10 minutes, according to size, until cooked. Serve with Cream and Parsley Sauce.
4. To serve cold, slip the trout into the boiling water, bring back to a boil, remove the pan from the heat, and leave to cool.
5. For the sauce, melt the butter in heavy pan.
6. When it has melted, stir in the cream. Keep stirring over a low heat until the sauce bubbles.
7. Season with salt and pepper and stir in the parsley. Serve at once.

Note: A green salad to which has been added some shredded Florence fennel root goes very well with the cold trout.

CHICKEN WITH LEMON

Serves 4–6

1 chicken (about 4 pounds)
4 tablespoons butter
1 lemon
1 onion stuck with a clove
1 sprig fresh tarragon (if not available, use parsley)
Sea salt
Freshly ground black pepper

1. Preheat the oven to 425°.
2. Clean the chicken and put half the butter inside the bird with a piece of lemon peel, the onion, the tarragon or parsley, a little sea salt, and freshly ground black pepper.
3. Squeeze the lemon and coat the outside of the chicken with the lemon juice, a little salt, and pepper.
4. Place the chicken on a large sheet of parchment baking paper* dotted with butter. Use the remaining butter to smear the breast and legs.
5. Pour over any remaining lemon juice and bring up the sides of the sheet of paper to enclose the chicken in a loose parcel. Enclose this in an outer sheet of aluminum foil. Do not seal too tightly.
6. Place in the oven and roast for approximately 1 hour.
7. Halfway through the cooking, remove the bird from the oven and baste thoroughly. Open the top of the parcel for the last 10 minutes to allow the breast to brown nicely.
8. This chicken is equally delicious served hot with green vegetables or cold with a green salad.

*The use of parchment baking paper prevents any possible aluminum contamination from the foil.

COLD CHICKEN À LA HAY

Serves 4–6

1 young chicken
1 bouquet garni (usually consists of
    2–3 sprigs parsley, 1 sprig thyme, 1
    bay leaf and 1 clove tied in a piece
    of muslin for easy removal)
2 egg yolks
1⅓ cups heavy cream
Grated peel of well-scrubbed lemon

1. Place the chicken in a large casserole dish with the bouquet garni, and half fill with water. Poach carefully in the oven at 350° until done. (The time will depend on the size of the chicken.)
2. Remove from the oven and allow to cool.
3. Divide the chicken into several large pieces and arrange on a serving dish.
4. Beat the egg yolks with the cream and stir over a low heat until slightly thickened, but do not allow to boil.
5. Pour over the chicken and sprinkle with the grated lemon peel. The sauce will thicken as the dish cools. Serve with a mixed green salad.

Variation

A delicious variation of this recipe is a simple tarragon chicken. Instead of using a bouquet garni when poaching the chicken, use several sprigs of fresh tarragon and, after the final dish has cooled, sprinkle the chicken with finely chopped fresh tarragon instead of lemon.

VEGETABLES WITH GROUND BEEF
Serves 3–4

2 teaspoons sunflower seed oil
12 ounces lean ground beef
Seeds from 3–4 cardamom pods
½ teaspoon dried thyme
1 small piece well-scrubbed orange peel
3 tablespoons water
2 cups mixed vegetables roughly chopped, such as 1 or 2 zucchini, 2 good-sized mushrooms, a large carrot, a piece of celery root, 3–4 shallots *or* 1 onion, ¼ red pepper (more if liked)
½ teaspoon potato flour
1 tablespoon finely chopped parsley
Sea salt and freshly ground black pepper

For garnish:

4–6 tomatoes
1 teaspoon chopped fresh basil (use dried basil if fresh not available)

1. Heat the oil in a heavy-bottomed pan. When medium-hot, add the ground beef, cardamom seeds, thyme, and orange peel and stir with a wooden spoon until all the meat grains are separated.
2. Add the water and prepared vegetables and cover the pan. Simmer at a very low heat for 1½ hours. Add a little more water during cooking if necessary, but when cooked the water should be nearly evaporated.
3. Mix the potato flour with 1 teaspoon water and stir into the mixture until it thickens slightly. Season and add the chopped parsley.
4. Turn onto a serving dish garnished with broiled halved tomatoes that have been sprinkled with the chopped basil.

INDIVIDUAL COLD SUMMER OMELETS*

To make one omelet

1 small tomato
1 large egg
Sea salt
Freshly ground black pepper
1 tablespoon butter
Chopped parsley

1. Skin, deseed, chop, and season the tomato.
2. Break the egg into a bowl and stir firmly with two forks, adding a mild seasoning of sea salt and freshly ground black pepper.
3. Warm a 6-inch omelet pan but don't make it too hot. Then turn the heat up to high.
4. Put the butter in the pan and when melted and just beginning to color, pour in the egg.
5. Add the tomato mixture and using a fork make sure it is folded well into the omelet.
6. From this point Elizabeth David's instructions cannot be bettered:

   Tip the pan toward you and with a fork or spatula gather up a little of the mixture from the far side. Now tip the pan away from you so that the unset egg runs into the space you have made for it. When only a little of the unset part remains on the surface the omelet is done. Fold it in three with your fork or spatula, hold the pan at an angle, and slip the omelet onto a plate.

7. Decorate with lots of chopped parsley.

Note: Cold stuffed omelets make a delicious salad meal, summer or winter. The stuffings can be varied: grated cheese, herbs, creamed mushrooms, or cooked peas.

*With grateful acknowledgment to Elizabeth David's *Summer Cooking* (Penguin Books).

SPANISH OMELET

Serves 2

4 teaspoons *plus* 1 tablespoon cold
pressed olive oil *or* sunflower seed
oil
1¾ cups prepared mixed vegetables,
such as sliced zucchini, a little
chopped red and/or green pepper,
chopped carrots, 1 or 2 sliced
mushrooms
1 tablespoon finely chopped parsley
Sea salt
Freshly ground black pepper
3 whole eggs *and* 1 yolk
¼ cup grated mild cheddar cheese

1. Heat 4 teaspoons oil in a heavy-bottomed pan.
2. Add the vegetables and stir for a few minutes over a medium heat until they start to give up their juices.
3. Turn the heat to very low and cook gently until tender but not mushy, stirring frequently.
4. At this stage, stir in the chopped parsley and season with salt and pepper.
5. Lightly beat the eggs and egg yolk and add the seasoning.
6. Preheat a 9-inch diameter omelet pan, add 1 tablespoon oil, and allow to become medium-hot (not smoking!).
7. Transfer the vegetable mixture to the omelet pan and spread evenly.
8. Pour the eggs onto the vegetable mixture and stir gently.
9. Continue to stir gently with a fork for half a minute or so until the omelet begins to set.
10. Top with the grated cheese and brown under a hot broiler. Do not allow the omelet to become too firm in the center.

11. Cut into two, loosen with a spatula, and slide onto a warmed serving plate.

Note: This is good with a green salad, watercress, or home-grown white mustard greens and garden cress.

STUFFED EGGS

Serves 4

    4 eggs
    Sea salt
    Freshly ground black pepper
    1 teaspoon yeast extract
    Yogurt
    Paprika
    Sprigs of parsley

1. Put the eggs into a pan of cold water, bring to a boil, and allow to boil for 10 minutes.
2. Pour off the water and allow the pan to stand under running cold water for a few minutes until the eggs are cold. (This prevents discoloration of the egg yolk).
3. Shell the eggs and cut in halves lengthwise.
4. Remove the yolks and place them in a blender or food processor, adding the seasoning and yeast extract. Blend with sufficient yogurt to make a stiff but creamy mixture.
5. With a teaspoon, neatly scoop out (and discard) some of the egg white in each half to enlarge the space for the filling.
6. Pile the egg yolk mixture into the scooped-out shells and decorate with a sprinkling of paprika and sprigs of parsley.

Note: This recipe can be made without a blender or processor by finely straining the egg yolk and then beating in the yogurt with an egg beater—but the processor gives a better result.

CHEESE SOUFFLÉ

For occasional use

Serves 2

1 whole egg *and* 1 yolk
1 cup milk
1 cup cubed cheese (mild cheddar)
1 medium-sized cooked and sliced
   potato
Sea salt
Freshly ground black pepper

1. Preheat the oven to 375°.
2. Place the egg, yolk, milk, and cheese in a blender and blend for a minute or so.
3. Add the sliced potato and seasoning and blend till all the ingredients are reduced to a smooth purée. (Potato is permissible here, as it is much less starchy than using flour for thickening.)
4. Divide the mixture into two buttered, oven-proof ramekins or soufflé dishes.
5. Bake for 30 to 35 minutes till golden brown on top, and serve immediately (they flop quickly!). Serve with Top Favorite All-seasons Salad (page 138).

CREAMED CAULIFLOWER CHEESE

Serves 4

1 medium cauliflower
1 cup cottage cheese
4 tablespoons heavy cream
½ cup grated cheddar cheese

1. Cut the cauliflower into thin slices and place in a thick-bottomed pan.
2. Add a little water and simmer gently over a low heat until the cauliflower is tender but not mushy and practically no water remains.
3. Using an egg beater or potato masher, beat the cauliflower in the pan to partly cream it.
4. Add the cottage cheese and enough cream to make a creamy mixture.
5. Turn into a shallow, greased baking dish, sprinkle with the grated cheese, and brown under the broiler.

ALMOND BALLS

Serves 4

1½ cups almonds
1½ cups additive-free cream cheese
A little crushed garlic (optional)
Toasted sesame seeds

1. Skin the almonds by dipping them into hot water to loosen the skins.
2. Chop the almonds and mix with the cream cheese.
3. Add the garlic if liked.
4. Shape the mixture into small balls and roll in the toasted sesame seeds.

Variation
This recipe can also be made with finely grated cheddar cheese in place of the cream cheese, by using a little cream to bind the mixture.

WHEAT GERM STUFFING

Can be used instead of the usual bread stuffings with roast chicken or turkey, or for stuffing potatoes.

> 4 heaping tablespoons wheat germ
> 2 tablespoons chopped parsley
> 1 large mushroom, finely chopped
> 1 tablespoon sunflower seed oil *or* melted butter
> 1 egg yolk
> 1 small onion, finely chopped
> 1 teaspoon lemon juice
> 1 heaping teaspoon dried thyme *or* 2 teaspoons fresh thyme
> 1 pinch dried marjoram
> Freshly grated nutmeg
> Sea salt
> Freshly ground black pepper
> Water, *or* dry red or white wine, to mix

1. Mix together the wheat germ, parsley, chopped mushroom, oil, egg yolk, onion, and lemon juice.
2. Add the herbs and a moderate grating of nutmeg.
3. Season and moisten with water or wine, as necessary.

FRUITY STUFFING

An excellent stuffing for chicken, lamb, or pork.

½ cup very sweet, dried apricots
¾ cup prunes
1 large apple
3 tablespoons wheat germ
½ cup freshly shelled walnuts, or
   other nuts of choice
Juice and grated rind of 1 well-
   scrubbed lemon
1 tablespoon cold pressed sunflower
   seed oil
1 egg yolk
Sea salt
Freshly ground black pepper

1. Blanch the apricots and prunes and soak overnight.
2. Cut the apricots and prunes into small pieces.
3. Peel the apple and chop it coarsely.
4. Chop the nuts, also rather coarsely.
5. Put all the ingredients into a bowl and mix thoroughly.

GRAVIES AND THICKENINGS WITHOUT FLOUR

To Thicken Gravies

Use potato flour. This is permissible as so little is required; one teaspoon or less is often sufficient. Mix 1 teaspoon of potato flour with a little cold water and stir into the meat juices and vegetable stock. Cook at a low heat as too-high heat makes the gravy go thin again.

To Thicken Stews

Cook the stew with plenty of vegetables and not too much water. When cooked, put some of the liquid from the stew or casserole with some of the vegetables in a blender and blend until thickened.

To Make a Coating Sauce for Vegetables

Mix an egg yolk into 2 tablespoons or more of heavy cream, season and add to the remaining vegetable juices in the pan in which the vegetables have been cooked (this should be reduced to 2–3 tablespoons) and cook gently over a low heat to avoid curdling. This coating is particularly good for carrots, zucchini, and snap and green beans. It not only enhances the taste of the vegetables but also makes use of the nutrient-rich vegetable water that is usually thrown away.

11.

VEGETABLES

RATATOUILLE

Serves 4

2 large onions
⅔ cup cold pressed olive oil
2 eggplants
2 red or green peppers
4–6 tomatoes

1. Peel and slice the onions.
2. Put the onions with the oil into a large, thick-bottomed pan over a low heat.
3. While the onions are softening, cut the unpeeled eggplants into cubes; remove seeds from the peppers and slice.
4. When the onions are soft, add the eggplants and peppers and allow to stew in the oil very gently for 10 minutes.
5. Peel and slice the tomatoes and add to the rest of vegetables. Continue to simmer with the lid on the pan for 30 minutes.
6. Take the lid off the pan and allow to simmer another 10 minutes.

Variation
This is a very flexible dish and quantities can be varied according to the availability of the ingredients. Zucchini can be substituted for the peppers if preferred, or if you have a glut in the garden.

ZUCCHINI DELUXE

Serves 4

8 medium zucchini
Sea salt
3–4 tablespoons heavy cream
Freshly ground black pepper
Finely chopped parsley

1. Wash the zucchini and slice into pieces ½-inch thick.
2. Pour into a heavy-bottomed pan with just sufficient water to cover the bottom of the pan.
3. Add a pinch of salt and the zucchini and cook at a moderate heat for 2 to 3 minutes, stirring constantly, until the skins become bright green.
4. Cover the pan and turn the heat to very low, adding a little extra water if necessary.
5. Simmer gently for about 6 minutes until the zucchini are tender but not mushy, stirring occasionally.
6. Remove from the heat and add the cream and a sprinkling of black pepper.
7. Let stand for a couple of minutes before serving, to allow the cream to thicken slightly and coat the zucchini.
8. Turn into a warm serving dish and garnish with chopped parsley.

Note: Using cream in this way is less fatty than the orthodox way of frying or sautéeing zucchini in butter or oil, in which they soak up an enormous quantity of fat in the cooking process.

BROCCOLI WITH LEEKS

Serves 4

1 pound broccoli
2 large leeks
½ teaspoon coriander seeds
Sea salt
Freshly ground black pepper
2 tablespoons virgin olive oil

1. Wash the broccoli and remove any tough stems and coarse or damaged leaves.
2. Steam the broccoli over boiling water until the stalks are just tender.
3. Wash and trim the leeks and cut across into slices.
4. Place the leeks in a pan containing 1–2 inches of boiling water to which you have added a little salt and the crushed coriander seeds.
5. Simmer gently for 4–5 minutes.
6. Remove the leeks from the water as soon as they are tender, drain, and place on a warmed serving dish.
7. Remove the broccoli from the steamer and arrange over the sliced leeks.
8. Dress with salt and freshly ground black pepper, and pour on the olive oil.
9. Serve hot or cold.

CELERY ROOT PUREÉE

Serves 4

Celery root, or celeriac, is a most useful vegetable and can be used to replace potatoes if you want a more substantial root vegetable to accompany meat or chicken dishes.

1½ pounds celery root
⅔ cup light cream
Sea salt
Freshly ground black pepper

1. Peel the celery root as thinly as possible, cut into even-sized pieces, and boil in lightly salted water until tender.
2. Drain the celery root and pass through a food mill, or mash by hand or in a food processor.
3. Return the celery root to the pan over a very low heat. Add the cream slowly, beating it into the purée thoroughly.
4. Season with sea salt (if needed) and freshly ground black pepper.

Note: This purée can also be served as a main course if topped with 1 cup grated cheddar cheese and placed under a hot broiler for a few minutes.

Variation
Parsnips can be prepared in the same way if celery root is not available.

BUTTERED CABBAGE

Serves 4

1 medium, firm cabbage
Sea salt
1 tablespoon butter
Freshly grated nutmeg
Freshly ground black pepper

1. Wash and shred the cabbage.
2. Put ¾ inch of water into a thick-bottomed pan, add a pinch of salt, and bring to a boil.
3. Add the shredded outer leaves of the cabbage, cover the pan, and boil for 3 minutes.
4. Add the rest of the cabbage and boil until the cabbage is cooked but still crisp (not more than 5 minutes).
5. Drain the cabbage, keeping the water for vegetable stock.
6. Rinse the pan, put in the butter, and melt over a medium heat.
7. Put in the cabbage with plenty of freshly ground black pepper and a little nutmeg.
8. Cover the pan and allow the contents to heat over a low heat for a minute of so, shaking or stirring the contents to mix them thoroughly. Serve at once so that the cabbage retains its crispness and nutty flavor.

SAVORY MUSHROOMS

Serves 4

12 medium to large, nicely cupped
  mushrooms
2 tablespoons butter
Sea salt
Freshly ground black pepper
Freshly grated nutmeg

1. Preheat the oven to 375°.
2. Wash and dry the mushrooms and place them, cup up-
   permost, in a lightly-buttered fireproof dish.
3. Put ½ teaspoon of butter into each cup.
4. Sprinkle each cup with a little salt, black pepper, and
   (most important) a little grated nutmeg.
5. Bake until well cooked; about 20 minutes.

Note: This is a delicious way of cooking mushrooms and
makes commercial ones taste almost like field mushrooms.

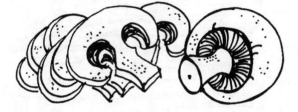

GARDENER'S SNAP BEANS

Serves 4

1 pound very small, young snap beans
1 tablespoon lemon juice
4 tablespoons heavy cream
2 tablespoons finely chopped parsley

1. Wash the beans and trim them, if necessary; if they are tiny, they will not need stringing or cutting.
2. Place in the top of a steamer and cook over boiling water until they are just tender.
3. Transfer the beans to a thick-bottomed pan over a medium heat.
4. Add the lemon juice and cream, and stir gently so that the beans are nicely coated.
5. Transfer to a warmed serving dish and sprinkle with the chopped parsley.
6. Serve at once.

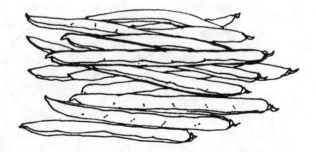

BUTTERED SPAGHETTI SQUASH

Serves 4

Spaghetti squash must surely be one of nature's greatest convenience foods. One plant will provide enough spaghetti squash to feed a family, so it is well worth giving up a corner of the garden to this unusual member of the squash family. When sliced, the inside flesh resembles threads of spaghetti—hence its name.

> 1 medium spaghetti squash
> 4 tablespoons butter
> Sea salt
> Freshly ground black pepper

1. Wash the spaghetti squash and prick the skin with a fork in two or three places.
2. Place in a steamer and steam over boiling water for about 45 minutes or until the flesh feels tender when pierced with a fork.
3. Remove from the steamer and place on a dish to drain.
4. Cut the spaghetti squash across into four thick slices and allow any water to drain away.
5. Place the slices on a warmed serving dish, season with a little salt and freshly ground black pepper, and place a pat of butter on each slice.
6. Serve at once.

Variation
Spaghetti squash can also be served as a main dish for two people if steamed as above, cut in half lengthways, and each half topped with ½ cup grated cheddar cheese. Finish by browning under the broiler.

12.

DESSERTS

FRUIT AND RASPBERRY DESSERT
For festive occasions

Serves 4–6

8 ounces frozen raspberries
4 large oranges
8 very sweet, dried apricots, soaked
  overnight
4 large ripe pears
⅔ cup sweet grapes
2–3 kiwi fruits
1 well-ripened banana

1. Defrost the raspberries and push through a fine nylon strainer.
2. Put the raspberry purée into a large mixing bowl with the juice of 2 of the oranges and some of the juice from the soaked apricots, so that the mixture has a creamy consistency, but is not thin.
3. Prepare the remaining fruit: peel the remaining oranges with a very sharp knife, removing the inner white pith along with the peel – the orange sections can then be removed whole and free of pith; cut the apricots into strips; peel, core, and slice one kiwi carefully and cut in thin slices; peel the banana and cut in slices.

4. Mix the prepared fruit into the raspberry sauce.
5. Turn the mixture into a suitable glass dish. Peel the remaining kiwis and cut carefully into thin rings. Mix the small end sections into the fruit mixture. Then arrange the kiwi rings in an overlapping circle on top of the dessert. This gives the dish an exotic appearance.
6. For a finishing touch, arrange a (clean!) half-opened pink rosebud upright in the center, or use any other suitable flower in season.

Note: The raspberry purée gives this dessert a beautiful color and delicious flavor. If the fruits are as sweet as they ought to be, no extra sweetening is necessary. When kiwis are not obtainable, a small handful of sun-dried raisins can be used instead, as a decoration.

Whipped cream can be served separately, if desired, but is not necessary.

FROZEN STRAWBERRY MOUSSE

Serves 2–3

2 cups defrosted frozen strawberries
    or fresh ones in season
2 tablespoons mild-flavored honey
⅔ cup heavy cream
2 rounded tablespoons non-instant
    skim milk powder, dissolved in
    very little water

1. Place the strawberries and honey in a blender or food processor and blend to a purée.
2. Whip the cream and dissolved milk powder until it stands in soft peaks.
3. Fold the strawberry purée into the cream.

4. Place in a suitable container or individual glasses, cover with aluminum foil, and freeze.

Note: This makes a delicious and very refreshing dessert for occasional use.

SPICED APPLE AND RAISIN PUDDING*

Serves 2–3

1 pound sweet eating apples
½ pound cooking apples
¾ teaspoon ground cloves
½ teaspoon ground cinnamon
⅔ cup raisins
¼ whole nutmeg, grated
1 tablespoon water

1. Core and peel the apples and slice thinly into a saucepan, adding the spices and raisins.
2. Sprinkle in the water and cook gently, with the lid on, for 10 minutes until the apples are soft and fluffy.
3. Serve either hot or cold (but it is especially good hot on a cold day, and a change from fresh, uncooked fruit).

Note: Made in batches of 3 pounds, this is an excellent way of using up windfalls and storing them in the freezer.
   By using mainly sweet eating apples, it should not be necessary to add sweetening.

*Adapted with grateful acknowledgment from the recipe for Spiced Apple and Raisin Pie in *Delia Smith's Cookery Course*, Part 1; one of Delia's many excellent recipes.

THREE QUICK APPLE DESSERTS

Baked Stuffed Apples

1. Wash and core one large eating apple for each person.
2. Fill the center of each apple with raisins or chopped dates. Place a teaspoon of honey over the filling.
3. Place in a baking dish and bake in a moderate oven (350°) — until the apples are tender — approximately 35–45 minutes.

Apricot and Apple Fool

Quantities can be varied according to the number of servings required.

1. Add one-third soaked, dried apricots to two-thirds cooked eating apples.
2. Place in a blender or food processor and blend to a thick but not too fine purée.
3. Add a little honey to taste and serve decorated with whipped cream and a sprinkling of chopped nuts.

Apple and Raisin Pudding

1. Place peeled and sliced eating apples, interlaced with raisins, in a baking dish and pour on the juice of one orange diluted with a little water.
2. Bake in a moderate oven (350°) until soft.
3. Sprinkle with a mixture of crushed nuts and wheat germ and serve with whipped cream. Good either hot or cold.

APRICOT MOUSSE

Serves 4

1½ cups dried apricots
4 tablespoons natural yogurt
Slivered almonds for topping

1. Wash and blanch the dried apricots and soak overnight in just enough water to cover them.
2. Place the apricots, with their juice, in a blender and blend until smooth.
3. Fold the yogurt into the apricot purée and pour into individual glasses.
4. Decorate with a topping of almonds.

Variation
For a richer dessert for special occasions, fold in ⅔ cup of whipped cream before pouring into the glasses.

NECTARINES IN A GLASS

Serves 4

4 really ripe nectarines
4 teaspoons mild clear honey
White wine, not too dry

1. Wash the nectarines well and dry carefully so that the skin is not damaged.
2. Do not peel them but, using a stainless-steel knife, slice each one straight into a wine glass. (To get the best effect, make the first incision down the natural division of the fruit from stalk to flower end. Slice out one section and continue slicing, turning the fruit as you cut, until all you have left is the pit.
3. Dribble 1 teaspoon of honey over each sliced nectarine and top each glass with white wine.

Note: Do not prepare too long in advance of the meal or the fruit may become sodden.

Variation
Peaches may be prepared in the same way but they should be peeled. In France, red wine is usually used to cover the peaches.

CHRISTMAS PUDDING

Serves 6–8

This is a favorite recipe with family and friends. It contains no flour or sugar and does not produce the "distended" feeling usually experienced after eating the traditional Christmas Plum Pudding.

> 2¼ cups seedless raisins (whole)
> 3½ cups seedless raisins (minced)
> 16 Santa Clara prunes, soaked for 2 days until soft, then pitted and minced
> ¾ cup finely chopped walnuts and almonds
> 1 cup prune juice (from soaking prunes)
> Juice of 1 large orange (and some grated rind if oranges are organically grown and therefore unsprayed)
> 2 cups ground almonds *or* freshly ground hazelnuts
> ½ cup brandy *or* whisky
> 2 egg yolks, well-beaten

1. Place all the ingredients in a mixing bowl and mix well.
2. Grease a 6 cup, oven-proof bowl and transfer mixture into it.

3. Cover the top with buttered waxed paper and an outer covering of foil.
4. Place bowl on a rack inside of a deep kettle; add an inch of boiling water to the kettle and replace kettle lid. Place kettle on a burner hot enough just to keep water at a slow boil.
5. Steam gently for 1 hour.
6. To serve, turn out carefully onto a warm serving dish, decorate with a piece of berried holly, pour a little brandy over the pudding, and ignite.
7. Can be accompanied with whipped cream, flavored with brandy.

Note: This pudding has a rich, fruity flavor, but if you prefer the traditional spicy flavor of Christmas pudding, one teaspoon of ground mixed spices can be added to the mixture.

This pudding will freeze satisfactorily for six weeks. Allow to thaw out gradually and steam for 45 minutes.

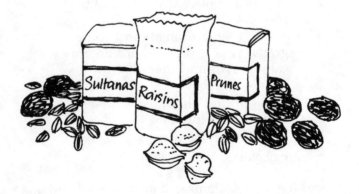

YOGURT

Makes one pint

Homemade yogurt is quick and easy to make. You need no special equipment apart from a wide-necked thermos bottle (also useful for transporting soup for sack lunches) and a cooking thermometer. If your family likes yogurt, you will save money by making your own.

> 2½ cups milk (whole milk *or* skim milk)
> 1 tablespoon non-instant powdered milk (optional)
> 1 teaspoon natural yogurt (as starter)

1. Put the milk into a thick-bottomed pan.
2. Whisk in the powdered milk if desired; it gives a better texture and thicker yogurt.
3. Heat the milk to 180° or to just below boiling point.
4. Cool the milk to 110° by placing the pan in a sink of cold water.
5. Rinse out the thermos with hot water. Pour most of the milk into the thermos.
6. Blend 1 teaspoon of natural yogurt with the remaining milk and add it to the thermos.
7. Twist the stopper on firmly and shake to mix well.
8. Leave for 4–6 hours or until firm.
9. Remove the stopper and put the thermos in the refrigerator to cool and set the yogurt.
10. You can use 1 teaspoon of this yogurt to "start" the next batch, but you will need a starter of fresh "live" yogurt every 7–10 batches.

Note: Here is another method of incubation:

1. Put the prepared milk in a lidded plastic container.

2. Wrap the container in a warm towel and leave it in a warm place, such as a gas oven with only the pilot light on.

Once made, the yogurt can be used in all the usual ways.
   For fruit yogurt, mix in the prepared fruit only *after* the yogurt has been made.

Pineapple Yogurt
Pineapple yogurt makes a quick and delicious dessert to follow a protein main course.
   Mix fresh, crushed, unsweetened pineapple with plain yogurt. Serve in individual bowls and sprinkle with sunflower seeds.

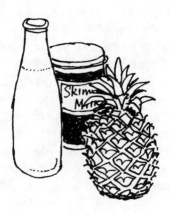

DINNER PARTY ICE CREAM
Serves 6

1⅓ cups heavy cream
1⅓ cups light cream
1 level tablespoon powdered milk
A little cold milk
1¾ cups chopped raisins
1¾ cups chopped cashews *or* other
   nuts
1 tablespoon maple syrup
2 teaspoons honey

1. Mix the creams together and beat until thick.
2. Mix the dried milk to a creamy consistency with a little cold milk and stir into the whipped cream.
3. Add the maple syrup and honey to sweeten, and then the chopped raisins and nuts.
4. Place the mixture in a suitable container, cover with aluminum foil, and freeze. Stir once during freezing.

Note: The addition of the dried milk powder is the secret of the success of this recipe; it prevents the ice cream from becoming hard and icy, and ensures a professional smoothness of texture. The ice cream will keep this texture even if kept in the freezer for a week or longer.

APRICOT SAUCE

1½ cups sweet, dried apricots
Juice of 1 large, fresh orange *or*
    diluted frozen unsweetened orange
    juice

1. Wash the apricots (blanch in boiling water and rinse again if the apricots are not organically grown).
2. Prepare the apricots by covering them with boiling water and soaking overnight.
3. Next day, place the apricots and some of the juice from soaking them in a blender. Add enough orange juice to make a sauce of medium thickness. It is difficult to be precise about quantities, but if you run the blender at low speed, you can add more orange juice until the sauce has reached the right consistency.
4. Serve as a dressing for peeled and sliced pears or other fruit. A little whipping cream makes a delicious addition to the sauce, giving it a smoother texture.

13.

PROTEIN SACK LUNCHES

There is no need always to think of sack lunches in terms of bread sandwiches. A protein meal is just as easy to transport.

A sack lunch can consist of leftover slices of cold meat or chicken, placed between lettuce leaves, or a chunk of cheese with a selection of celery sticks, raw carrots, slices of fresh fennel root, sprouts, tomatoes, cucumber chunks, green or red pepper rings, or chunks of fresh coconut. To finish, pack any of the acid fruits, such as apples, pears, and oranges. If still hungry, sunflower seeds make a delicious filler, and on cold days the meal can be preceded by a hot vegetable soup carried in a thermos.

Another good sack lunch consists of Individual Cold Omelet (page 160) accompanied by lettuce, sprouts, or other salad vegetables, followed by fresh fruit.

PART FOUR
RECIPES FOR STARCH MEALS

14.

SOUPS

CELERY ROOT SOUP

Serves 4–6

1 onion
2 celery roots, weighing in total
    about 1½ pounds
4 tablespoons butter
3¾ cups vegetable stock
Sea salt
Freshly ground black pepper
4 tablespoons light cream
Chopped fresh parsley

1. Peel and chop the onion, peel the celery root, and cut it into cubes.
2. Melt the butter in a heavy saucepan and cook the onions gently for 2–3 minutes. Add the celery root and cook for another 5 minutes, stirring constantly.
3. Add the stock, bring to a boil, cover the pan, and simmer until the celery root is tender.
4. Pour the soup into a blender and blend until smooth.
5. Return it to the pan, add seasoning, and reheat.
6. Stir in the cream and serve with plenty of chopped parsley.

POTATO SOUP

Serves 4

1 leek
2 tablespoons butter
4 potatoes, about ½ pound each
2½ cups vegetable stock *or* water flavored with ½ teaspoon yeast extract
Sea salt
Freshly ground black pepper
Grated nutmeg *or* 1 teaspoon curry
  powder

1. Wash the leek thoroughly and slice.
2. Melt the butter in a thick-bottomed pan and add the chopped leek. Allow to cook gently without coloring.
3. Add the potatoes, peeled and quartered, and the vegetable stock.
4. Bring to a boil, cover the pan, and simmer gently until the potatoes are tender.
5. Place in a blender and blend until smooth.
6. Return the soup to the pan, season with salt and pepper, and add a little milk or more stock if preferred, to give a creamier consistency.
7. Lastly, add a pinch of nutmeg or a teaspoon of curry powder.
8. Reheat and serve, sprinkled with chopped parsley.

MIXED VEGETABLE SOUP

Serves 4–6

½ pound parsnips
½ pound carrots
½ pound rutabaga or turnips
2 celery stalks
4 tablespoons butter
5 cups vegetable stock
1 teaspoon yeast extract
Sea salt
Freshly ground black pepper
Freshly chopped parsley

1. Cut all the root vegetables into smallish slices and chop the celery.
2. Melt the butter in a heavy pan, add the root vegetables, and cook them gently for about 5 minutes.
3. Add the vegetable stock, yeast extract, and chopped celery and bring to a boil. Turn down the heat and simmer gently for about 10 minutes until the vegetables are tender but not mushy.
4. Place in a blender and blend for a few seconds so that the texture is thick but still fairly coarse.
5. Return the soup to the pan and reheat; season with salt and pepper.
6. Serve with a good sprinkling of chopped parsley.

Note: If you grow herbs and have a lovage plant, the addition of *one* leaf of lovage improves the flavor of this soup.

ASPARAGUS SOUP

Serves 4

This soup can be made from asparagus stalks — the tips being served as a vegetable in the usual way.

> 2 pounds asparagus
> 1½ cups chopped onion
> 3 tablespoons butter
> 2 teaspoons potato flour
> 2 cups asparagus stock (from cooking tips and stalks)
> Sea salt
> Freshly ground black pepper
> 1 tablespoon chopped parsley
> 2 tablespoons heavy cream

1. Cook the asparagus — tips and stalks — in the usual way. Serve the tips as a vegetable. Reserve the stalks and the asparagus stock.
2. In a thick-bottomed pan, melt the butter, add the chopped onion, and sauté the onion until it is golden.
3. Add the asparagus and stock and simmer for about 10 minutes to extract the full flavor.
4. Purée the liquid in a blender and strain to remove any stringy pieces.
5. Return the soup to the pan and add the potato flour, which has been mixed to a smooth paste with a little water.
6. Add the seasonings to taste and heat until just below boiling point.
7. Add the parsley, stir in the cream, and serve.

15.

SALADS

POTATO SALAD

Serves 4

4 large *or* 8 small new potatoes
2 celery stalks
2–3 scallions
2 tablespoons light cream
Sea salt
Freshly ground black pepper
3–4 fresh mint leaves

1. Cook the potatoes in their skins.
2. While still warm, remove the skins and let potatoes cool.
3. Dice the potatoes, chop the celery and scallions, and mix together.
4. Dress the salad with the cream, seasoned with salt and pepper and flavored with chopped mint leaves.

Note: Leftover waxy potatoes can also be used to make this salad.

BROWN RICE SALAD

Serves 4

1 cup long grain brown rice
3 cups water
1 level teaspoon sea salt
3 scallions, chopped finely
1 red pepper, deseeded and sliced
  finely
½ cup seedless raisins
½ cup coarsely chopped pecans
1 tablespoon olive oil
Salt and freshly ground black pepper
  to taste
A little chopped fresh parsley

1. Put the rice into a strainer and pour cold water through it to remove any dirt.
2. Put the rice and water in a large pan and bring to a boil.
3. Boil for 1 minute, cover the pan, and turn the heat down so that the water is barely simmering.
4. Cook for about 40 minutes, then test. The grains should be chewy, but not mushy.
5. Drain the rice in a colander and rinse it with cold water. Set it aside until cool.
6. While the rice is cooking and cooling, prepare the remaining ingredients.
7. When the rice is almost cold, add the onions, pepper, raisins, and nuts.
8. Pour oil over the salad and toss well, adjusting seasoning if necessary.
9. Place the salad in a serving dish and garnish with chopped parsley.

TABOULI

Serves 6

1 cup bulghur (cracked wheat)
3 tablespoons finely chopped scallions *or* 1 onion, finely chopped
Salt and freshly ground black pepper
6 tablespoons parsley, finely
  chopped
3 tablespoons fresh mint, finely
  chopped
4 tablespoons olive oil
2 tablespoons grated rind of a well-
  scrubbed lemon
Lettuce
1 green pepper

1. Soak the bulghur in water for about ½ hour. Drain and press out as much moisture as you can with your hands. Spread out on paper towels to dry still further.
2. Mix the bulghur with the chopped onion, turning thoroughly to allow the juices to penetrate the grains. Season to taste with salt and pepper.
3. Add the parsley, mint, olive oil, and lemon rind and mix well. Taste to find out whether more seasoning or lemon is needed. There should be a distinct lemony flavor.
4. Pile onto a large serving dish lined with crisp lettuce leaves and strips of green pepper.

PECAN AND PASTA SALAD

Serves 4

2 cups whole wheat pasta shells
1 green pepper, deseeded
¾ cup pecans
⅓ cup raisins
4 tablespoons Sour Cream Dressing
   for starch meals (page 205)

1. Cook the pasta in boiling salted water until just tender.
2. Drain well and allow to cool.
3. Chop the green pepper finely and mix with the pasta.
4. Add the pecans and raisins.
5. Mix well with the Sour Cream Dressing and serve.

Note: This salad is substantial enough to be served as a main dish. If used as a side dish, the portions should be smaller and this quantity would serve 6–8.

FAVA BEAN AND SAVORY SALAD

Serves 4

2 pounds young tender broad beans
2–3 sprigs summer savory
White mustard greens and garden
   cress
⅔ cup sour cream
Sea salt
Paprika

1. If the bean pods are really small and tender, simply wash, top, and tail them and cut into short lengths. If larger, shell the beans.
2. Put the beans into *just* enough boiling water to cover

them, add a pinch of salt and a sprig of savory, and cook with the lid on the pan until they are just tender (10–15 minutes).

3. Drain the beans and allow to cool.
4. Arrange on a bed of white mustard greens and garden cress and dress with the sour cream, which has been seasoned with a pinch of paprika and a teaspoon of finely chopped savory leaves.

CARROT AND RAISIN SALAD

Serves 4

⅓ cup seedless raisins
1½ cups grated raw carrot
Lettuce
3 tablespoons light cream
Sea salt
Freshly ground black pepper

1. Soak the raisins in water for a couple of hours before making the salad.
2. Mix the grated carrot with the soaked raisins and arrange on a bed of lettuce.
3. Season the cream with salt and pepper and pour over the grated carrots.

BANANA AND DATE SALAD

The quantities for this salad will vary according to the number of people to be served.

> 1 small banana per person
> Grated or very finely chopped nuts
>   *or* toasted sesame seeds
> 1 head of lettuce or other greens
> 4 dates per person
> ½ cup additive-free cream cheese
> About ¾ cup light cream
> 1 teaspoon clear, mild honey
> Fresh mint leaves *or* freshly grated
>   rind of a well-scrubbed lemon

1. Cut the banana into quarters and roll the pieces in the grated nuts or toasted sesame seeds.
2. Wash and dry the lettuce leaves and arrange on a serving dish to form a base for the other ingredients.
3. Arrange the banana pieces on the bed of lettuce.
4. Remove the pits from the dates, fill the centers with cream cheese, and arrange on the dish.
5. Dress the salad with the cream, sweetened with a teaspoon of honey, flavored with a pinch of freshly chopped mint leaves or a little grated lemon rind.

EGGPLANT PÂTÉ

Serves 4

3 large eggplants
1 clove garlic
2 tablespoons olive oil
*1 tablespoon lemon juice
Sea salt and freshly ground black
   pepper
**2 teaspoons chopped fresh tarra-
   gon if available

1. Preheat the oven to 350°.
2. Place the eggplants in a shallow baking dish and bake
   in the oven for about 45 minutes.
3. Remove the eggplants from the oven and allow to cool
   slightly. Cut in halves and remove the flesh; put this
   through the medium disk of a food mill.
4. Add the crushed garlic and stir in the olive oil and
   enough of the lemon juice to sharpen the purée.
5. Add salt and pepper to taste, stir in the chopped tarragon, and put into a dish.
6. Chill thoroughly before serving.
7. Serve on whole wheat toast as a light meal or in smaller
   quantities as an appetizer. This will freeze but is better
   fresh.

*Permissible because so little is used.
**If no tarragon is available, decorate the pâté with a little
finely chopped parsley before serving.

SALAD DRESSINGS FOR STARCH MEALS

Cooked vegetable salads can be dressed simply with a little seasoned olive oil. The best oil for salads and cooking is cold-pressed virgin olive oil. As this is now so expensive and it is often difficult to find a really good tasting one, cold-pressed sesame oil and sunflower seed oil are the best alternatives.

Non-acid French Dressing

Use equal parts of fresh raw tomato juice and olive or sunflower seed oil. Season with sea salt, paprika, and any fresh herbs available. Fresh chopped tarragon or basil are very good additions.

Simple Cream Dressing

Add sea salt, freshly ground black pepper, and any fresh chopped herbs available to ⅔ cup light cream. Good with mixed shredded raw vegetable salads.

Avocado Cream Dressing

Blend the flesh of one ripe avocado with a little light cream and season with sea salt and paprika. Very good with a mixed green salad.

Egg Yolk Topping

Egg yolks are a rich source of vitamins and minerals. Hard boil the eggs, chop the yolks finely (or press through a strainer), and season lightly with sea salt. Use as a decorative and nutritious topping for salads and vegetable dishes.

Sour Cream Dressing

   ⅔ cup sour cream
   Freshly grated rind of a well-
    scrubbed lemon
   Sea salt
   Freshly ground black pepper
   1 teaspoon clear, mild honey (op-
    tional)

1. Mix all of the ingredients well before pouring over the
salad. This dressing is best prepared just before serving.

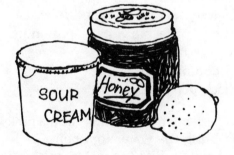

16.

MAIN DISHES

SPAGHETTI WITH PESTO SAUCE

Serves 4

8 ounces uncooked, whole wheat
   spaghetti
Sea salt

For the pesto sauce:

1 large handful chopped fresh basil
¾ cup pistachio nuts *or* pine nuts
6 large tomatoes
½ cup olive oil
Black pepper

1. Half fill a large pan with water, add a tablespoon of sea salt, and bring the water to a boil.
2. Put the spaghetti into the water, pushing it down into the pan as it softens.
3. Simmer gently for about 10 minutes until the spaghetti is just tender but still has a bite to it—"al dente."
4. Drain the spaghetti well and slide it into a well-oiled and heated dish.
5. While the spaghetti is simmering, make the pesto.
6. Peel the tomatoes, chop coarsely, and place in a blender.

7. Add the basil, nuts, salt and pepper, and the olive oil.
8. Blend everything together and adjust the seasoning if necessary.
9. Pour the pesto over the spaghetti, add a little butter, and toss the spaghetti well. Serve at once.

PASTA SHELLS WITH PARSLEY SAUCE

Serves 4

2 cups whole wheat pasta shells
Sea salt
For the parsley sauce:
2 tablespoons butter
¼ cup whole wheat flour
1⅓ cups milk
2–3 tablespoons chopped parsley
Sea salt
Freshly ground black pepper

1. Place the pasta shells in a pan of boiling water with a pinch of sea salt and cook for 10–12 minutes or until "al dente" (just cooked but not soggy).
2. In a heavy pan, melt the butter and stir in the flour. Stir with a wooden spoon until the mixture bubbles.
3. Remove the pan from the heat and slowly add the milk, stirring all the time to prevent lumps forming.
4. Return to the heat and stir constantly until the sauce thickens and has reached the boiling point.
5. Wash and chop the parsley and add to the sauce.
6. Drain the pasta and place on a serving dish.
7. Reheat the sauce and pour over the pasta. Serve with a green salad.

RICE WITH LEEKS AND CASHEWS

Serves 4

1 cup long grain brown rice
3 cups water
4 large *or* 6 small leeks
2 tablespoons butter
⅓ cup seedless raisins
⅓ cup cashews

1. Put the rice and water into a pan (one that has a lid) and bring to a boil; boil fiercely for 5 minutes, then cover and turn the heat down. Simmer for 40 minutes.
2. Put the butter into a thick-bottomed pan and melt gently. Add the leeks, which have been thoroughly cleaned and cut into thin rounds by slicing across the stems.
3. Cover the pan and turn the heat down so that the leeks cook gently in their own liquid until tender, but still crisp. Be careful not to overcook. The green part of the leek should remain bright green. 5–10 minutes is usually long enough for this process but the time varies a little according to the thickness of the leeks.
4. When the leeks are done, transfer them to a colander to drain, return to the pan, and add the raisins and cashews.
5. When the rice is done, mix the contents of the two pans together and test for seasoning, adding a little sea salt and ground black pepper if necessary, and serve.

RICE PILAFF

Serves 4

2 cups mixed raw vegetables—choose
  from: peas, carrots, celery, leeks,
  red or green peppers, or celery
  root
2 tablespoons butter
Dried mixed herbs
Sea salt
Freshly ground black pepper
*1½ cups cooked brown rice
½ cup raisins
½ cup chopped nuts
1 teaspoon curry powder (optional)

1. Prepare the raw vegetables; dice the carrots and celery or celery root, and slice the leeks and peppers.
2. Place the prepared vegetables (except the peas) in a heavy pan with the butter.
3. Cook gently over a low heat for about 10 minutes, stirring frequently.
4. Add just enough water to cook the vegetables without their sticking to the pan, a pinch of dried mixed herbs, salt and pepper. For variety, add a teaspoon or so of curry powder as soon as the carrots are cooked.
5. Cook the peas in a separate pan to retain their color.
6. When the vegtable mixture is tender and thick in consistency, add the rice, raisins, and peas, and chopped nuts.

*To Cook Brown Rice

For every cup of brown rice allow 3 cups of water. Put the rice and water into a thick-bottomed pan (one with a tightly fitting lid) and bring to a boil. Boil for 5 minutes, then cover the pan and turn the heat down as low as you can so that the water is barely simmering. Simmer for 40 minutes. Do not stir while cooking. When the rice is tender, the water should have been completely absorbed, but if there should be any left, drain the rice and return to the pan for a few minutes to dry off before serving.

VEGETABLE CASSEROLE
Serves 4

2 tablespoons butter
3 onions, peeled and sliced
2½ cups carrots, scrubbed and sliced
2½ cups potatoes, peeled and sliced
2 celery stalks, washed and chopped
1 green pepper, washed, deseeded, and cut into strips
3 cups button mushrooms, washed and sliced
2½ cups water *or* vegetable stock
1 tablespoon tomato paste
1 large bay leaf
2 teaspoons potato flour
Sea salt
Freshly ground black pepper

1. Preheat the oven to 375°.
2. Melt the butter in a heavy frying pan and sauté the onions until golden. Add the rest of the vegetables and continue to cook for another 2–3 minutes, stirring often.
3. Transfer to a flameproof casserole dish and add the water or stock, tomato paste, bay leaf, and seasoning.
4. Bring the contents of the casserole to a boil, then transfer to the oven and cook for 45 minutes.
5. Remove from the oven and add the potato flour, which has been mixed to a smooth paste with a little water. Stir well, adjust the seasoning, and return to the oven for another 15 minutes.

HAZELNUT ROAST

Serves 4

2 cups hazelnuts
4 cups whole wheat bread crumbs
1⅓ cups chopped onion
1⅓ cups grated carrot
Sea salt
Freshly ground black pepper
½ teaspoon dried mixed herbs
2 egg yolks
A little milk

1. Preheat the oven to 375°.
2. Chop the hazelnuts coarsely.
3. Mix the nuts, bread crumbs, onion, and carrots together well.
4. Add salt and pepper to taste, and the dried herbs.
5. Add the beaten egg yolks and, if necessary, a little milk to bind the mixture.
6. Place in a well-greased loaf pan and bake for 45 minutes. Serve with a cooked green vegetable or a green salad.

POTATOES DAUPHINOIS À LA HAY

Serves 2

2 baking-sized waxy new potatoes
  per person
1 small onion per person (or adjust
  quantity according to taste)
Sea salt
Freshly ground black pepper
A little heavy cream *or* about 1 tablespoon butter

1. Scrub the potatoes well to remove the outer thin brown skins and cut into thin slices. Preheat the oven to 425°.
2. Coarsely chop up the onions.
3. Place an inch or so of water in a thick-bottomed pan, and add the chopped onion and sliced potatoes.
4. Season lightly with sea salt and freshly ground black pepper.
5. Cook over a moderate heat for 6–8 minutes, until the potatoes are nearly cooked and there is only a little water left in the pan.
6. Turn the contents of the pan, including the valuable potato water, into a shallow, buttered ovenproof dish.
7. Arrange the potato slices to make a nice flat surface and dribble over it some heavy cream, or dab all over with a piece of butter.
8. Bake for about 30 minutes or until the potato slices on top are golden brown and becoming crisp.

Note: This is an excellent and very savory main course for a starch meal, accompanied with a salad or vegetables, or with white mustard greens and garden cress. Cooked this way, potatoes are economical as far as fat (butter or cream) is concerned, compared with "Potatoes Anna" or to baked potatoes, which tempt one to overdo the butter. (This recipe is now so popular with my husband that he prefers it to any other way of cooking potatoes.)

This dish can also be made with old potatoes, but the skins will then have to be removed, *as thinly as possible*, with a vegetable peeler.

POTATO AND LEEK HOTPOT

Serves 2

2 medium leeks
2 tablespoons butter
1½ pounds potatoes
1 cup water
Sea salt
Freshly ground black pepper
2 tablespoons heavy cream
Chopped parsley

1. Clean and slice the leeks.
2. Melt the butter in a heavy-bottomed pan and add the sliced leeks.
3. Cook over a low heat, stirring frequently until the leeks are a light golden color.
4. Pare and slice the potatoes and add them, with the water, to the leeks.
5. Cook over a very low heat, stirring occasionally, till the potatoes are cooked and almost sticking to the bottom of the pan—this gives the hotpot its excellent flavor! If the mixture becomes at all dry, add a little more water.
6. Add the seasoning and stir in the cream just before serving. Sprinkle with chopped parsley for decoration.

BAKED POTATOES WITH MUSHROOM FILLING
Serves 4

4 medium potatoes of uniform shape
and sound skins
A little sunflower seed oil
½ cup hot milk
1 tablespoon butter
Sea salt
Freshly ground black pepper
Freshly grated nutmeg

For the mushroom filling:

4 cups open mushrooms
6 tablespoons milk
2 teaspoons potato flour
Grated nutmeg
½ teaspoon yeast extract
2 tablespoons heavy cream

1. Preheat the oven to 400°.
2. Scrub the potatoes well, prick with a fork, and smear the skins with sunflower seed oil.
3. Bake in the oven for 1 hour, or until the skins are crisp.
4. Cut potatoes in two, remove the flesh, and return the skins to the oven to keep crisp.
5. Mash the potato flesh well in a pan with the milk and butter to make a light creamy mixture.
6. Season to taste with salt, black pepper, and especially the nutmeg.
7. Refill the potato shells with the mixture, making a hollow in the centers with the back of a spoon to hold the mushroom filling.
8. Clean the mushrooms and slice thinly.
9. Cook gently in the milk for about 10 minutes until tender.
10. Mix the potato flour with a little cold milk and add to the mushrooms to thicken.

11. Season to taste, add a grating of nutmeg (this has a magical effect on the flavor of the mushrooms), the yeast extract, and the cream.
12. Fill the potato hollows, and reheat and brown them under the broiler. Serve with a green salad or with white mustard greens and garden cress.

BAKED POTATOES WITH CREAM CHEESE AND HERBS

Serves 4

4 medium potatoes
1 cup cream cheese
2 tablespoons yogurt
1 pinch sea salt
1 pinch paprika
Chopped chives, tarragon, savory, or
  any other fresh chopped herbs

1. Preheat the oven to 350°.
2. Scrub the potatoes thoroughly but do not peel.
3. Score once lengthways across the upper side of each potato and bake for 30–40 minutes.
4. While the potatoes are baking, mix the cream cheese with the yogurt and add salt, paprika, and chopped herbs to taste.
5. Remove the potatoes from the oven and arrange them on a serving dish. Put the cream cheese mixture into a pastry bag and pipe over the slit in the baked potatoes.

BAKED POTATOES WITH CRISPY SKINS

Allow one medium-sized potato per person. Using a sharp knife, score slits across the back of the potato about ⅛ inch apart. Season the slits and rub butter over them. Bake in the oven for about 40 minutes at 350°.

An unusual and delicious way of baking potatoes.

POTATO CAKES

Serves 4

1½ pounds potatoes
4 tablespoons light cream
1 egg yolk
1 pinch sea salt
¼ teaspoon grated nutmeg
1 tablespoon chopped marjoram
1 tablespoon chopped chives

1. Scrub the potatoes and steam or boil them in their skins until cooked.
2. Drain the potatoes and remove their skins.
3. Mash thoroughly with the cream and egg yolk, adding salt to taste, the nutmeg, and the herbs.
4. Form the mixture into patties and bake them on a greased baking sheet in a hot oven (425°) until slightly browned. Serve with a mixed vegetable salad.

Variation
Use 2 tablespoons of sunflower seeds and 2 tablespoons of chopped parsley instead of the chives or marjoram.

VEGETABLES

Most of the main dishes based on grains or potatoes in this section are fairly substantial and need only a green salad, dressed with a little olive oil, or some home-grown white mustard greens and garden cress, to accompany them.

If, however, a side dish of cooked vegetables is required, it is best to serve one or two green vegetables that have been conservatively cooked, either in just a little water (keep the liquid for vegetable stock), or better still, steamed. A good steamer with dividers, so that more than one vegetable can be cooked at the same time, produces delicious vegetables that retain all their natural flavor, and is very economical to use. Pressure cookers are not recommended for green vegetables; they tend to overcook, however carefully they have been timed. All vegetables lend themselves to steaming and the larger ones can be sliced or chopped before cooking to shorten the cooking time.

The following vegetables are particularly good steamed:

• Asparagus tips (keep the stalks to make Asparagus Soup—page 196)

• Tiny brussels sprouts, served with a little butter and topped with slivered almonds

• Young green or snap beans

• Broccoli

• Spring carrots

• Sliced eggplant

• Celery, cut into short lengths to steam and served with a little butter

• Cauliflower flowerets

• Small onions steamed whole, or larger ones sliced

• Fresh garden peas, steamed with a sprig of mint and served with butter

- Sliced parsnips, steamed and served with a little butter
- Spaghetti squash or any other type of squash

Any leftover vegetables prepared in this way retain plenty of flavor and can be incorporated into a vegetable soup the next day.

17.

DESSERTS

BANANA CREAM

Serves 4

> 2 large *or* 3 small bananas
> ⅔ cup natural yogurt
> ⅔ cup whipping cream
> Sunflower seeds

1. Blend the bananas in a blender and mix well with the yogurt.
2. Whip the cream until stiff and fold into the banana mixture.
3. Serve in individual bowls topped with a scattering of sunflower seeds.

DATE ICE CREAM

Serves 4

16 pitted dates
1 cup water
1 tablespoon non-instant powdered
   skim milk
⅔ cup whipping cream

1. Put the dates in a blender. Add the water and powdered milk and blend until smooth.
2. Whip the cream until stiff and fold into the date mixture.
3. Place in a container, cover with foil, and freeze until firm.
4. Remove from the freezer, beat with a fork to ensure a smooth texture, and refreeze.

GINGER BANANAS

Serves 4

4 ripe bananas
A little preserved ginger
Slivered almonds

1. Slice the bananas into individual dishes (one per person).
2. Rinse the syrup from the preserved ginger and chop fairly finely.
3. Sprinkle ginger over the bananas and top with a few almonds. Serve with a little whipped cream.

Variation
Another way to serve bananas is to slice them as above, mix in a few drops of lemon juice (permissible because so little is used) to stop them going brown, and sprinkle with sunflower seeds.

EGG CUSTARD

Serves 2

¾ cup milk
2 egg yolks
Mild honey to taste
A few drops of *real* vanilla extract
(optional)

1. Heat the milk to boiling point and add slowly the well-beaten egg yolks.
2. Return to the pan, preferably a double boiler, and stir over a gentle heat until the mixture thickens slightly.
3. Sweeten to taste with a mild-flavored honey and add a few drops of vanilla extract if liked. The custard will thicken as it cools.

Variation
Make an egg custard as above. With kitchen scissors, snip dried figs into thin slices. Place in individual bowls and sprinkle on some finely chopped preserved ginger (any sugar adhering to the ginger can be washed off), allowing a scant teaspoon per serving. Top with the custard and decorate with whipped cream and/or chopped nuts of choice.

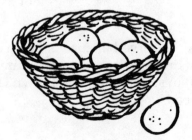

MORE DESSERT IDEAS FOR STARCH MEALS

- Sliced *fresh* figs in season—good alone or with a little thin cream

- Fresh dates, stuffed with freshly shelled walnuts

- Dried date chips

- Very sweet ripe pears, sliced and served with a little light cream

- Frozen bananas. Simply peel one banana per person and put in the freezer as it is. When frozen solid, remove and put in the refrigerator for half an hour. Serve with a sprinkling of nuts and you have banana ice cream!

- Baked pears with raisins. Peel and halve very ripe pears. Place in a baking dish with a scattering of raisins and a little water. Bake at 350° for about 20 minutes.

18.

BREAD

This book would not be complete without giving the recipe for the delicious and easy no-kneading Grant loaf.

Since it was first published in *Your Daily Bread*, it has introduced countless families to the pleasure of eating really good whole wheat bread. It has also acquired a few variations, which are included here.

You will not, however, find any recipes for cakes or cookies as they have no place in the Hay system except for *very* occasional use. For the occasional indulgence, the authors heartily recommend *The Cranks Recipe Book* by David Canter, Kay Canter, and Daphne Swann, which contains excellent sections on cakes, scones, cookies, and bread, and many other mouth-watering recipes for soups, salads, and main dishes that can be adapted for the Hay system.

For people who are allergic to gluten, *The Sunday Times Book of Real Bread* gives many good bread recipes that offer a healthy alternative to the whole wheat loaf, and Hilda Cherry Hill's book *Good Food Gluten Free* offers many helpful recipes and ideas for coping with gluten allergy. A more recent book, *Cook Yourself a Favor* by Sheila L.M. Gibson, Louise Templeton, and Robin G. Gibson, offers practical suggestions for following wheatless diets and many delicious recipes for using oats, barley, rye, and other grains.

Note: All the following bread recipes freeze well.

THE GRANT LOAF

For three loaves

12 cups stone ground, whole wheat
flour
2 teaspoons or less sea salt
5 cups water at (98°) body temperature
3 level teaspoons dried baking yeast
2 level teaspoons brown sugar,
honey, or blackstrap molasses

1. Mix the salt with the flour (in very cold weather, warm the flour slightly to take off the chill).
2. Place 3 tablespoons of the water in a cup, sprinkle the dried yeast on top, and leave for 2 minutes.
3. Add the sugar, honey, or molasses. Let stand for 10–15 minutes, by which time there should be a thick creamy froth.
4. Make a well in the center of the flour and pour in the yeast mixture and the rest of the water.
5. Mix well — by hand is best — for a minute or so, working from sides to middle until the dough feels elastic and leaves the sides of the mixing bowl clean. Flours tend to vary in how much water they take up — the dough should be slippery.
6. Divide the dough into three 5-cup bread pans, which have been warmed and greased.
7. Put the pans in a warm (not hot) place, cover with a clean cloth, and leave for about 20 minutes or until the dough is within ½ inch of the top of the pans.
8. Bake in a fairly hot oven (400°) for 35–40 minutes. If the loaf sounds hollow when the top is tapped, it is done.

For one loaf

- 4 cups stone ground, whole wheat flour
- ½ teaspoon sea salt
- 1¾ cups water at (98°) body temperature
- 1½ level teaspoons dried baking yeast
- 1 teaspoon brown sugar, honey, or blackstrap molasses.

The Bran-plus Loaf
In the Grant Loaf recipe, substitute ⅓ cup fresh unprocessed bran for ⅓ cup whole wheat flour in every 4 cups.

The Gordon Grant Loaf
In the Grant Loaf recipe, substitute ¼ cup medium oatmeal for ¼ cup whole wheat flour in every 4 cups. Before baking the loaves, sprinkle sesame seeds thickly on top of the dough and press them down gently to make them adhere.

Note: The oatmeal enhances the lovely nutty flavor of the bread and increases its moisture-keeping quality.

Oven Whole-wheat Flatties
Save some of the dough when making Grant loaves. Place heaping tablespoons of dough on to a greased baking sheet, leaving ample room between them. With floured hands, press the mounds of dough into flat rounds – as flat as you can make them. Allow to rise until nicely puffed, then bake for about 20 minutes at bread temperature until they are pale golden brown on top and crisp underneath.

The flatties can be eaten as soon as they are cold; consisting mainly of a well cooked crust, they are not indigestible like new bread can be. To serve, slit them open horizontally, remove any doughy inside, butter both halves, and fill with various mixtures, such as egg and sprouts, honey and chopped parsley, or lettuce with a mixture of chopped fresh herbs. They are delicious eaten soon after they are cool, but not good if kept till the next day.

OATCAKES

> 1 cup medium oatmeal
> ½ cup boiling water
> ½ level teaspoon sea salt
> 1 level teaspoon unsalted butter

1. Preheat the oven to 350°.
2. Put the oatmeal into a mixing bowl.
3. Using a Pyrex container, pour the boiling water over the sea salt and unsalted butter to melt them, add to the oatmeal, and mix well.
4. Let stand for a minute or so, until the oatmeal swells and becomes workable.
5. Turn the mixture onto a well-floured pastry board and form into two equal-sized balls.
6. Roll out each ball separately into a small round and then cut this across four times to make eight wedge-shaped pieces.
7. Roll out each wedge as thinly as possible, rolling from cut edge to cut edge—not from the outer edge to the point—in order to make nicely shaped pieces.
8. Place the cakes on a baking sheet and bake them until the wedges are slightly curved and a light golden color. When cool, store in an airtight container.

Note: These oatcakes are delicious and quite different from factory-made ones. Make sure that the oatmeal smells, and tastes, really *fresh*. Stale oatmeal tastes slightly bitter.

COOKED OATMEAL

Serves 2

1 cup medium oatmeal
2½ cups water
1 pinch sea salt

1. Bring the water to a boil in a thick-bottomed pan.
2. Stir in the oatmeal and cook at just under boiling point for 3 minutes, until it starts to thicken.
3. Add the sea salt to taste and pour into bowls. As it cools slightly, the oatmeal will thicken to the right consistency.
4. Serve with milk or cream.

Note: It is a good idea to sprinkle the cooked oatmeal with raw oatmeal just before serving. This ensures that the porridge is well chewed rather than just swallowed – chewing is very important for starch digestion.

SANDWICH FILLINGS FOR SACK LUNCHES

Use a genuine whole wheat bread such as the Grant loaf, or whole wheat rolls, which are quicker and easier to prepare than cutting sandwiches.

Suggestions for fillings:

- Mashed dates with grated lemon or orange rind
- Dates and chopped celery
- Dates and roughly chopped walnuts
- Sliced tomatoes and lettuce leaves with chopped chives
- Sliced cucumber and sprouts
- White mustard greens and garden cress with savory butter (butter flavored with a little yeast extract) or sesame seed spread
- Sprouts with cottage or cream cheese—but not a hard cheese such as cheddar; even the soft cheeses constitute a compromise
- Mashed bananas with chopped cashews or almonds
- Cream cheese with chopped fresh herbs
- Mashed banana with chopped fresh parsley
- Cold scrambled egg yolks with sprouts
- Mashed cooked peas with a little chopped mint
- Any available mixed salad greens with savory butter
- Cold snap beans mashed with chopped hard-boiled egg yolk

Any of the above sandwiches preceded by a thermos of hot vegetable soup and followed by a handful of nuts and raisins or sunflower seeds would make an excellent and sustaining meal.

APPENDIX
ACID AND ALKALI-FORMING FOODS

A balanced diet consists of 20 percent acid-forming foods and 80 percent alkali-forming foods.

The Acid-forming Foods
Meat (all kinds), including meat broths, extracts, and soups
Poultry and game
Fish (all kinds) and shellfish
Cheese
Eggs
All grains – wheat, rice, oats, barley, buckwheat, and grain products, except millet
Bread (all kinds)
Breakfast cereals (all kinds)
Flours of all kinds, especially white flour
Sugar of all kinds and all products containing it; e.g., jams and preserves, cookies, pastries, soft drinks, cola drinks, and commercial ice cream
Beans; e.g., broad, navy, kidney, and soy beans
Peas (dried)
Legumes; e.g., lentils, chick peas (garbanzos), peanuts, and peanut butter (not recommended)
Walnuts, cashews, and pecans

Note: Whole grain products such as 100 percent whole wheat flour and brown rice are less acid-forming than white flour or polished rice. Condiments, pickles, sauces, and vinegar are all acid-forming as well as tea, coffee, and alcohol. Seeds such as sunflower, sesame, and pumpkin may be regarded as neutral.

Dairy Products
*Milk — preferably raw — *not boiled or pasteurized.*
Buttermilk
Yogurt
Kefir
Fresh cream
Cream cheese

*Milk is a food for young mammals and should always be used sparingly by adults. It should be regarded as a food, not a drink, and should not be served at a meal containing meat. It should be used only in moderation with cereals and starches.

When heat treated, milk becomes more or less acid-forming according to the degree of heat supplied.

Fats
Butter and vegetable oils such as olive, sunflower seed, safflower, and sesame seed oils are regarded as neutral.

The Alkali-forming Foods

Fruits	*Vegetables*
Apples	Asparagus
Apricots (fresh or dried)	Avocados
Bananas	Beets
Cherries	Broccoli
Currants — red, black or white, *if ripe*	Brussels sprouts
	Cabbages — all types
Dates	Carrots
Figs (fresh or dried)	Cauliflower
Gooseberries *if ripe*	Celery
Grapefruits	Celery root
Grapes	Chives
Kiwis	Cucumbers
Lemons	Dandelion leaves

Fruits (continued)
Oranges
Mangoes
Melons
Nectarines
Papayas
Peaches
Pears
Pineapples (fresh)
Prunes—Santa Clara prunes
  only
Raisins—all kinds
Raspberries
Strawberries

Nuts
Almonds
Brazil nuts
Chestnuts
Hazelnuts
Pine nuts (pignolias)

Grains
Millet

Vegetables (continued)
Eggplants
Endive
Fresh green peas
Kale
Kohlrabi
Leeks
Lettuces
Mushrooms
Mustard greens and garden
  cress
Onions
Parsnips
Peppers, green and red
Potatoes in skins
Radishes
Rutabagas
Scallions
Sea vegetables
Spinach
Spring greens
Squash
String beans
Tomatoes
Turnips
Watercress
Zucchinis

FURTHER READING

General
Peptic Ulcer, T.L. Cleave (John Wright & Sons Ltd., 1962).
The Role of Medicine: Dream, Mirage or Nemesis, Thomas McKeown (Nuffield Prov. Hosp. Trust, 1976).
The Diseases of Civilisation, Brian Inglis (Hodder & Stoughton, 1981).
Cured to Death – The Effects of Prescription Drugs, Arabella Melville & Colin Johnson (Secker & Warburg, 1982).
Health Shock, Martin Weitz (David & Charles, 1980).
Living Dangerously, Hilda Cherry Hills (Tom Stacey, 1973).
Cover Up – The Facts They Don't Want You to Know, Nicholas Hildyard (New English Library, 1981).
Diet, Crime and Delinquency, Alexander Schauss (Parker House, 1980).
Health and Light, John Ott (The Devin Adair Co.).
The Western Way of Death, Dr. Malcolm Carruthers (Davis-Poynter, 1974).
Food for Nought – The Decline in Nutrition, Ross Hume Hall (Harper & Row, 1974).
Food Additives and Your Health, Beatrice Trum Hunter (Keats Publishing Inc., 1972).
Pure, White & Deadly, The Problem of Sugar, John Yudkin (Davis-Poynter, 1972).
Dieting Makes You Fat, Geoffrey Cannon & Hetty Einzig (Century Publishing, 1983).

Physiology of Gastric Digestion, A.M. James (Arnold, 1957).
The Work of the Digestive Glands, Ivan Pavlov (Charles Griffin & Co. Ltd., 1910).

Health and Nutrition

Food Combining Handbook, Gary Null and Staff (Berkley Publishing Group, 1983).
Sugar Blues, William Dufty (Warner Books, Inc., 1975).
Fit for Life, Harvey and Marilyn Diamond (Warner Books, Inc., 1985).
Food Combining Made Easy, Herbert M. Shelton (Willow Publishing, 1985).
The Yeast Connection, William G. Crook, M.D. (Vintage Books, 1986).
Nutrition and Health, Sir Robert McCarrison & H.M. Sinclair (McCarrison Society, 1982).
The Saccharine Disease, T.L. Cleave (John Wright & Sons Ltd., 1974).
Dietary Fibre, Refined Carbohydrate Foods and Disease, Dr. Hugh Trowell (Academic Press, 1984).
Don't Forget Fibre in Your Diet, Dr. Denis Burkitt (Martin Dunitz, 1979).
Taking the Rough with the Smooth, Dr. Andrew Stanway (Pan, 1981).
A New Health Era, Dr. William Howard Hay (Harrap: out of print but second hand copies may be obtainable from secondhand book shops).
Your Daily Food — Recipe for Survival, Doris Grant (Faber & Faber, 1973).
The Food and Health of Western Man, Dr. James Lambert Mount (Charles Knight, 1975).
Everything You Should Know About Your Food, Claire Loewenfeld (Faber & Faber, 1978).
The Right Way to Eat, Miriam Polunin (J.M. Dent & Sons Ltd., 1978).
Know Your Nutrition, Linda Clarke (Keats Publishing Inc., 1973).

The Pritikin Program for Diet & Exercise, Nathan Pritikin and Patrick M. McGrady Jr. (Bantam, 1980).
The Joy of Beauty, Leslie Kenton (Century Publishing, 1983).
Man Alive, You're Half Dead!, Dr. Daniel Munro (Bartholmew House Inc. 1957).
Your Diet in Health and Disease, Harry Benjamin (Thorsons, 1974).
Foods for Health and Healing, Dr. Dudley d'Auvergne Wright (Health Science Press).
Natural Weight Control, N.W. Walker (O'Sullivan Woodside & Co., 1981).

Allergy and Related Problems
Why Your Child is Hyperactive, Dr. Ben F. Feingold (Random House, 1975).
Not All in the Mind, Richard Mackarness (Pan, 1976).
Chemical Victims, Richard Mackarness (Pan, 1980).
Eating and Allergy, Robert Eagle (Thorsons, 1986).
My Ivory Cellar, John Ott (Twentieth Century Press, Inc. 1958).
The Treatment of Asthma, Dr. Harrington (M.K. Lewis & Co. Ltd., 1936).

Eating for Health; Wholefood Cookbooks
Confessions of a Sneaky Organic Cook, Jane Kinderlehrer (Rodale Press Inc., 1971).
The Cranks Recipe Book, David Canter, Kay Canter, & Daphne Swann (Thorsons Publishers, Inc., 1985).
Eating Naturally, Maggie Black & Pat Howard (Faber & Faber, 1980).
Food Naturally, Sue Bennett (W.H. Allen, 1979).
Health Food Cookery, Marguerite Patten (Hamlyn, 1972).
High Fibre Cooking, Janette Marshall (Thorsons, 1983).
The High Fibre Cookbook, Pamela Westland (Martin Dunitz, 1982).
Jane Grigson's Vegetable Book (Penguin, 1980).
Sugar Off!, Richard & Elizabeth Cook (Great Ouse Press, 1983).

The Sunday Times Book of Real Bread, Michael Bateman & Heather Maisner (Rodale Press Inc., 1982).
A White Eagle Lodge Book of Health & Healing, Joan Hodgson (White Eagle Publishing Trust, 1983).

Vegetarian Cookbooks
Any books by Rose Elliot, but in particular:
   Gourmet Vegetarian Cooking (Fontana, 1983).
   Not Just a Load of Old Lentils (Fontana, 1983).
   Simply Delicious (Fontana, 1981).
   Your Very Good Health (Fontana, 1981).
The Bircher-Benner Health Guide, Ruth Kunz-Bircher (George Allen & Unwin, 1981).
Eating Your Way to Health, Ruth Bircher & Claire Loewenfeld (Faber & Faber, 1966).
The Bristol Diet, Dr. Alec Forbes, Medical Director of the Cancer Help Centre (Century Publishing, 1984).
The Four Seasons Wholefood Cookbook, Susan Thorpe (Thorsons, 1983).
Gail Duff's Vegetarian Cookbook (Pan, 1979).
The Vegetarian Epicure, Anna Thomas (Penguin, 1973).
The Vegetarian Gourmet, Judy Ridgeway (Ward Lock, 1979).

Macrobiotics
The Book of Whole Meals, Annemarie Colbin (Ballantine Books, 1983).
Cook Yourself a Favour: 350 Recipes to Help You Help Yourself to Better Health, Sheila L.M. Gibson, Louise Templeton, & Robin Gibson (Thorsons, 1986).

Vegan
Healthy Eating for the New Age, Joyce d'Silva (Wildwood House, 1980).
What Else is Cooking?, Eva Batt (Vegan Society Ltd., 1983).

Raw Foods, Herbs, and Salads
Raw Energy, Leslie & Susannah Kenton (Century Publishing, 1984).

The Raw Food Way to Health, Janet Hunt (Thorsons, 1978).
Herbs for Health & Cookery, Claire Loewenfeld & Philippa Back (Pan, 1965).
A Herb Cookbook, Gilian Painter (Hodder & Stoughton, 1983).
The Home Herbal, Barbara Griggs (Jill Norman & Hobhouse, 1982).
Stay Slim with Herbs & Spices, Elizabeth Peplow (Darton, Longman & Todd, 1981).

Growing Your Own
Culinary and Salad Herbs, Eleanor Sinclair Rohde (Dover Publications Inc., 1972).
The Salad Garden, Joy Larkcom (Windward, 1984).
Salads the Year Round, Joy Larkcom (Hamlyn, 1980).

Directories: Where to Find Wholefood and Organic Suppliers
The Cook's Lifeline, Joy Montague (Exley Publications, 1983).
International Vegetarian Handbook 1983/4 (The Vegetarian Society, Parkdale, Dunham Road, Altrincham, Cheshire).
The Organic Food Guide, Edited by Alan Gear (Henry Doubleday Research Association, 1983).

Note: All the cookbooks listed above contain excellent recipes that can be adapted to the Hay System and are particularly helpful in providing new ideas for the preparation of salads, fruits, and vegetables.

In case of difficulty, most of them can be obtained from the Wholefood Bookshop, 24 Paddington Street, London W1M 4DR, England; or see the list of publishers under "Useful Addresses."

Useful Addresses

Food and Supplements for Exclusion and Special Diets
For information about local whole food and organic suppliers consult: *The Organic Network*, edited by Jean Winter, published by Eden Acres, Inc., 1984. Updated annually. Available from: Eden Acres, Inc., 12100 Lima Center Road, Clinton, Michigan 49236. Tel. (517) 456-4288.

Mailorder Services for Whole Foods and Organic Supplies:
Walnut Acres, Penns Creek, Pennsylvania 17862. Tel: (717) 837-0601.
The Good Food Store, 920 Kensington, Missoula, Montana 59801. Tel: (406) 728-5823.
Eden's Foods, 701 Tecumseh Road, Clinton, Michigan 49236. Tel: (517) 456-7424.
Kahan and Lessin Distributors, 3131 E. Maria Street, Compton, California, 90221. Tel: (213) 631-5121.

Teas, Herb Teas, Herbs, and Spices
Aphrodesia Products, 45 Washington Street, Brooklyn, New York 11201.
Biobotanica Inc., 75 Commerce Drive, Hauppauge, New York 11788.
Green Mountain Herb, Inc., 4890 Pearl Street, Boulder, Colorado 80301.
San Francisco Herb, Tea and Spice Trading Company, 4543 Horton Street, Emeryville, California 94601.
Sweethardt Herbs, Box 12602, Austin, Texas 78711.
The Whole Herb Company, 250 East Blithedale, Mill Valley, California 99494.

In Canada:
Lifestream, 12411 Volcan Way, Richmond, BC, Canada V6V 1J7.
Wide World of Herbs, 11 Saint Catherine Street East, Montreal 129, Canada.

Organic Honey Suppliers
Draper's Super Bee Apiaries, RD 1, Box 97, Millerton, Pennsylvania 16936. Tel: (800) 233-4273.
Francis and Elizabeth Bradac, Ramblewood Acres, 985 Englewood Avenue, St. Paul, Minnesota 55104.

Allergy, Hyperactivity, and Nutrition
Allergy Foundation of America, 801 2nd Avenue, New York, New York 10017. (Fosters research in allergic reactions to food.)
International College of Applied Nutrition, PO Box 386, La Habra, California 90631. (Specializes in nutritional aspects of disease.)
National Academy of Sciences, 2101 Constitution Avenue NW, Washington, DC 20418. Tel: (202) 334-3318. (Up-to-date information on additives, disease, and nutrition).
Food and Drug Administration, Public Health Service, Department of Health, Education and Welfare, 5600 Fishers Lane, Rockville, Maryland 20857. Tel: (301) 443-3170.

Publishers
Academic Press, 111 Fifth Avenue, New York, New York 10003.
Allen, W.H. & Company PLC, 44 Hill Street, London W1X 8LB, England.
American Medical Publishing Association, PO Box 1900, Santa Barbara, California 93102.
BBC Publications, 35 Marylebone High Street, London W1M 4AA, England.
Ballantine Books, Inc., 201 E. 50 Street, New York, New York 10022.
Bantam Books, Inc., 666 Fifth Avenue, New York, New York 10103.
Bartholomew House, John & Son, Inc., c/o Herman Publishing, Inc., 45 Newbury Street, Boston, Massachusetts 02116.
Berkley Publishing Group, Jove Books, 200 Madison Avenue, New York, New York, 10016.
BMA House, Tavistock Square, London WC1H 9JR, England.
British Diabetic Association, 10 Queen Anne Street, London WM1M OBD, England.
Century Publishing Company Ltd., 76 Old Compton Street, London W1, England.

Charles Griffin & Company Ltd., Crendon Street, High Wycombe HP13 6LE, England.

Clinic for Alternative Medicine, Lane End, Highlands Lane, Westfield, Woking, Surrey GU22 9PU, England.

Darton, Longman & Todd Ltd., 89 Lillie Road, London SW6 1UD, England.

David & Charles Ltd., Brunel House, Newton Abbot, Devon TQ12 4PU, England.

Davis-Poynter Ltd., 11 Bolt Court, Fleet Street, London EC4A 3DQ, England.

Dent, J.M. Ltd., 33 Welbeck Street, London W1M 8LX, England.

Deven-Adair Company Publishers, 143 Sound Beach Avenue, PO Box 1, Old Greenwich, Connecticut 06870.

Doubleday, Henry Research Association, 32 Convent Lane, Bocking Braintree, Essex England.

Dover Publications, Inc., 180 Varick Street, New York, New York 10014.

Edward Arnold Publishers Ltd., 41 Bedford Square, London WC1B 3DQ, England.

Exley Publications Ltd., 16 Chalk Hill, Watford, Herts WD1 4BS, England.

Faber and Faber, Inc., 39 Thompson Street, Winchester, Massachusetts 01890.

Fontana Paperbacks, 14 St. James Place, London SW1A 1PF, England.

Fontana, John M., Publisher, 4 Walnut Place, Huntington, New York 11743.

George Allen & Unwin Publishers Ltd., 40 Museum Street, London WC1A 1LU, England.

Great Ouse Press, 62 Castle Street, Cambridge CB3 OAJ, England.

Grosset & Dunlap Inc., 51 Madison Avenue, New York, New York 10001.

Hamlyn Publishing Group Ltd., Astronaut House, Hounslow Road, Feltham TW14 9AR, England.

Harper & Row Publishers, 10 E. 53 Street, New York, New York 10022.

Harrap Ltd., 19023 Ludgate Hill, London EC4M 7PD, England.

Health Education Council, 78 New Oxford Street, London WC1A 1AH, England.

Health Science Press, 1 Church Path, Saffron Walden CB10 1JP, England.

H.K. Lewis & Company Ltd., 136 Gower Street, London WC1E 6BS, England.

Hodder & Stoughton Ltd., 47 Bedford Square, London WC1B 3DD, England.

Homeopathic Development Foundation Ltd., 19A Cavendish Square, London W1M 9AD, England.

Homeopathic Trust Royal London Homeopathic Hospital, Gt. Ormand Street, London WC1N 3HR, England.

Houghley Soil Association, Walnut Tree Manor, Haughley Stowmarket LP14 3RS, England.

Jill Norman, Rosslyn Hill, London NW3, England.

John Wright & Sons Ltd., 42-44 Triangle West, Bristol, BS8 1EX, England.

Johnston Green Publishing Group, PO Box 1, Portree, Isle of Skye 1V1 9BT, England.

Keats Publishing, Inc., 27 Pine Street, PO Box 876, New Canaan, Connecticut 06840.

Martin Dunitz Ltd., 154 Camden High Street, London NW1 ONE, England.

McCarrison Society Publications, 76 Harley Street, London W1N 1AE, England.

Medical News-Tribune Ltd., 359 Strand, London WC2R OHP, England.

New American Library, University of South Carolina, English Department, Columbia, South Carolina 29208.

New England Journal of Medicine, 10 Shattuck Street, Boston, Massachusetts 02115.

New English Library, Mill Road, Dunton Green, Seven Oaks, Kent TN13 2YA, England.

Nuffield Provincial Hospital Trust, 3 Prince Albert Road, London NW1 7SP, England.

O'Sullivan, Woodside & Company, 2218 Magnolia, Phoenix, Arizona 85034.

Pan Paperback, Pan Book Ltd., 18-21 Cavaye Pls., London SW10 9PG, England.

Parker House, 2340 Parker Street, Berkeley, California 94704.

Penguin Books, 625 Madison Avenue, New York, New York 10022.

Penguin Publishing, PO Box 23196, Rochester, New York 14692.

Random House, Inc., 201 E. 50 Street, New York, New York 10022.

Roberts Publications, 225-229 Putney Bridge Road, London SW15 2PY, England.

Rodale Press, Inc., 33 E. Minor Street, Emmous, Pennsylvania 18049.

Royal College of General Practitioners, 14 Princes Gate, Hyde Park, London SW7 1PU, England.
Royal Society of Medicine, Proceedings of the, Chandos House, 2 Queen Anne Street, London W1M OBR, England.
Secker & Warburg Ltd., 54 Poland Street, London W1V 3DF, England.
Stacey International, 128 Kensington Church Street, London W8 4BH, England.
Stacey Publications, 1 Hawthorndene Road, Hayes, Bromley B52 7DZ, England.
The Lancet, 7 Adam Street, Adelphi, London WC2N 6AD, England.
Thorsons Publishers, Inc., Park Street, Rochester, Vermont 05767.
Times Newspapers Ltd., Gray's Inn Road, PO Box 7, London WC1 8EZ, England.
Twentieth Century Press, Inc., John Ott Publisher, 1873 Hillview Street, Sarasota, Florida 33579.
Vegetarian Society, Parkdale, Dunham Road, Altrincham, Cheshire, England.
Ward Lock Ltd., 82 Gower Street, London, WC1, England.
Warner Books, Inc., 666 Fifth Avenue, New York, New York 10103.
Which Business Publications Ltd., 20A Camberwell Green, London SE5 7AA, England.
White Eagle Publishing Trust, New Lands, Brewell Lane, Liss GU33 7HY, England.
Wildwood House Ltd., Gloucester Mansions, Cambridge Cirus, Charing Cross Road, London WC2H 8HD, England.
Willow Publishing, Inc., San Antonio, Texas
Windward Publishing, Inc., 105 NE 25 Street, PO Box 371005, Miami, Florida.

Index

244 *Food Combining for Health*